I HAD BEEN SO FOCUSED ON JAKKI, I HAD IGNORED THE OTHERS.

Now, hands grabbed me from behind. I reached for my bludgeon, but one of them nimbly unhooked it.

"Hit her!"

"Kill her!"

"She betrayed us! She will lead the Guards here!"

Shrill voices cried out in vindictive fear.

"No." Jakki motioned to whoever was behind me. "Tie her up. Take the jacket and shoes. We can sell them, use the coin for food. We will not kill her—it is wrong to kill. We will let the river spirits do with her what they will." He pointed to the cave's exit. "Put her under the bridge. We will let the tide take her away."

ALSO BY ROBERTA ROGOW

THE SAGA OF HALVAR THE HIRELING

Murders in Manatas
Mayhem in Manata
Mischief in Manatas
Menace in Manatas
Malice in Manatas
Madness in Manatas

THE POLA DRACH MYSTERIES

Lorr and Disorder

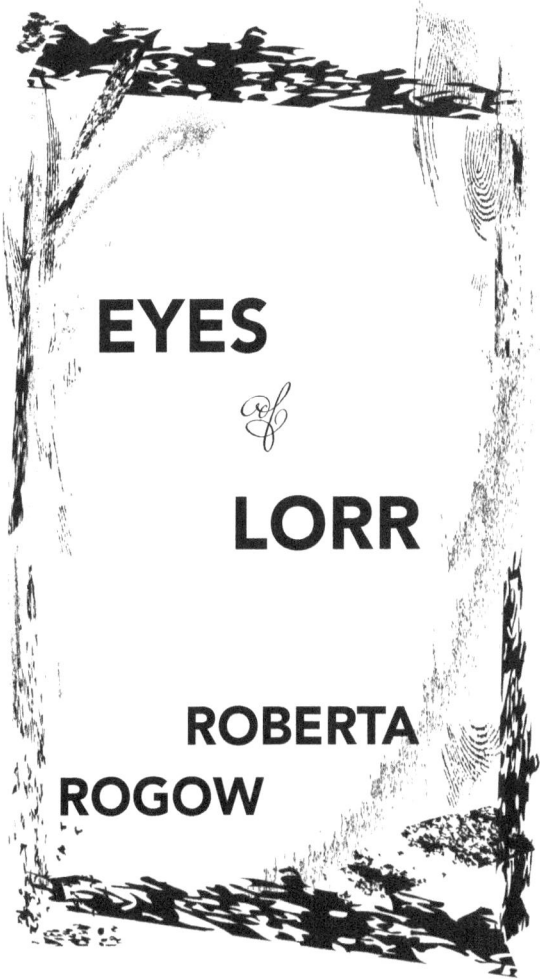

EYES

of

LORR

ROBERTA ROGOW

ZUMAYA OTHERWORLDS   AUSTIN TX

2021

EYES OF LORR
© 2021 by Roberta Rogow
ISBN 978-1-61271-391-5
Cover art and design © Jennifer Givner

"Zumaya Otherworlds" and the griffon colophon are trademarks of Zumaya Publications LLC, Austin TX
https://www.zumayapublications.com

Library of Congress Control Number: 2021941167

TO JACQUELINE LICHTENBERG AND JEAN LORRAH

Who introduced me to the marvelous world of fan fiction many years ago

NOTES FOR SALE

IT ALL BEGINS WITH THE CLIENTS.

They come to me with their problems, and ask me to solve them. Usually, it's personal, not something for their Guild Security to bother with, and definitely not something that would draw the City Guard into their orbit. A spouse that's cheating, a family member taking advantage of an elderly parent, a child gone missing.

They come to the little room behind Jake and Holly's Boutique, they tell me what they want me to do. I find out what they need to know, I tell them, and they go ahead and do what they feel has to be done.

I'm Pola Drach, Independent Eye. I'm not directly connected with any of the Guilds. I'm not in the Guards. I have no political affiliation. I just watch and listen, and report.

My clients are mostly Middle Tier Lorrans, what you might call above-the-below and below-the-upper. Small shopkeepers, office drones, mechanics, and technicians. Sometimes refugees from the religious bickering in Pangkot, come to Lorr for work and safety, or Norlanders who've had their fill of ice and snow. Once in a while I get a bigger fish, someone connected with the Upper Tier families. I've even done a job for Master Assassin Fee M'Farr…but that's a story for another time.

This client was definitely not from Lorr. He was Contramonti, from the toes of his lizardskin boots to his flat-crowned straw hat. Nice, bland face, nothing to distract, no obvious scars or odd features—just regular eyes, nose, mouth all adding up to a good-looking whole, but nothing to distinguish him from anyone else in Lorr. Blue eyes took in my spare quarters, reddish-blond hair sticking out from under the hat. Reddish-blond fuzz sprouted from his square chin—too young, then, to grow a full beard like the Contamonti Elders.

Wearing the standard Conty garb—blue cotton trou held up with straps attached to a bib across his chest worn over a full-sleeve blue shirt, braided cord keeping the shirt closed at the neck. Broad shoulders, good solid chest, well-built under the baggy outfit. In other words, a typical youngster fresh from the countryside, ready to take in the perils and delights of the City of Lorr.

He hesitated as he came in the door, as though worried he was doing the right thing, coming to me. I don't look like much—medium height, medium weight, honey-gold skin, fair hair, green eyes, just the far side of thirty.

I was wearing one of my autumn outfits of a brown jacket, yellow shirt, brown trou. Nothing gaudy, nothing too worn. I wouldn't be noticed in a crowd. That's the way I like it, and it works for my clients.

I smiled, encouraging him to come in. "Oyo, how's business? What brings you here, friend?"

"I'm Zacharias Garber, I'm here in Lorr with the Contramont Miners' trade delegation," he stated in passable Lorr Standard, flavored with the distinctive Conty twang. "I've lost something. I need to have it back, quickly. I was told you are the one who finds things."

I looked him over while he stood shifting from foot to foot.

"Sit down, and tell me about it."

He plumped himself into the wooden chair across the desk from mine. It's deliberately uncomfortable. I don't want clients lingering, chattering, wasting my time when I could be getting on with the job.

He shifted in his seat. "The…the persons on Entertainment Row said you would help me."

Persons? Either buskers or the Licensed sex workers who walk the street, trolling for customers. I'd have to find out which one pointed him in my direction. It's a debt, and in Lorr, all debts have to be paid.

"I'll do my best to help you." I reached into the drawer next to the kneehole in my desk and pulled out one of my standard contracts and the graphite stylus I keep handy for clients. "What did you lose? When did you see it last? And what do you want me to do when I find it?"

"It's my notebook," he burst out. "I've got to find it! It's got everything in it—all my thoughts and feelings, all my work notes. I keep it here." He patted his chest. "Inside my bib pocket."

"Did you take it out and leave it somewhere?"

"No, no. It must have fallen out when…"

He stopped. A blush started somewhere under his chin and spread across that fair face.

"You took off your trou," I said slowly. "On Entertainment Row? In one of the Pleasure Houses?" I didn't have to ask how or why. It was obvious, written on his red face.

"It was a party," he went on. "I didn't think I should go, but Elder Mackintosh said it was an obligation, since it was arranged by the Banker's Guild representative, the one who was in favor of promoting our funding. Elder Mackintosh was quite insistent that we accept their hospitality, even though it might be somewhat..." He paused. "I didn't know quite what was involved in such an affair. I thought it would just be food and drink. I didn't expect the...other entertainment."

Meaning Licensees. I got the picture. Get the Contramonters muzzy, ply them with jack and spray weed around; then turn the Licensees loose to pick up whatever they could wangle out of them. Standard operating technique for merchants in Lorr, where anything goes if it brings in a profit. I'd have thought better of the Banker's Guild, but everyone has their off-moments.

"So, you went," I said. "And you accepted the hospitality offered."

"I did," Friend Zac moaned. "I had no idea it would be that kind of place...that kind of party..."

"Not the sort of thing they do in Contramont," I finished for him.

Beyond the mountains, folks get prudish, clinging to the Second Ship customs that separate genders. Especially true in Contramont, where things get downright rigid when it comes to male-female relationships.

4

"So, you were lured into a bedroom by one of the wicked females, removed your trou…"

Zacharias's blush turned purple. "Not a female," he whispered. "His name was Emil. I'd never, ever thought I would…that is, I wanted…but it's a sin, I mustn't…" He stopped, gripped by shame.

"I'm not here to judge you," I said with a confidential smile. "What happens in Lorr stays in Lorr. I assume you and this Emil are both over puberty, and the encounter was part of the entertainment, paid for in advance by whoever was throwing this, um, party. And that no force was involved on either side."

It doesn't matter to me whether the two parties involved are male or female or mixed. No one in Lorr cares what anyone does in private with anyone else, so long as it's consensual, and both parties are over puberty.

Nonconsensual intimacy is another matter—that's rape, in any language or dialect, and it's the one thing in Lorr that will bring every law-enforcement organization down on the perpetrator in force. The City Guard won't stand for it; the Entertainment Guild won't turn their backs on it; even the Fatsos—the Honorable Guild of Forgers, Assassins, Thieves, and Swindlers—draw the line there. The Regs don't cite many things as "crime" in Lorr, but rape is right up there with unsanctioned killing and running out on a debt.

Zac nodded, the blush fading from his cheeks.

"There was no force. I went upstairs willingly with Emil. It was…enlightening.

"Then, there was noise downstairs. Emil helped me put on my overalls, and we went down. There was some kind of disruption going on—some other people had come into the place, large men in leather jackets who demanded attention. Our host protested, said he had paid for access for the entire evening. The intruders were very rude.

"Then a squad of City Guards came in, said they had been notified there was a riot in the making. There were words exchanged, and the person in charge made everyone leave. Pedi-shaws were summoned to take us to our lodgings. I left with the others, back to the Stranger's Hostel at the Advanced Academy, where I have a room.

"I do not know how I got into bed, but someone else must have been there. I fell asleep. And in the morning, when I woke, I realized the book was gone."

"And you went back to Entertainment Row?"

He nodded. The purple of embarrassment was replaced by the pallor of terror.

"I tried to recall which of the places was the one we visited, but they all look alike in the dark, and by daylight I couldn't remember which one it was. And then one of the…the persons…on the street told me to go to Clothier's Alley and talk to Pola Drach."

I appreciated his delicacy of language. Most Contys would have called them "women"or, worse,"whores".

"Well, Friend Garber…"

"Call me Zac."

"Friend Zac, here are my terms. I charge a silver a day. For this, I will find your missing book, and return it to you. You understand that if I find out something that goes against the Regulations of the City of Lorr, I have to report it to the City Guards."

"You've been listening to those people who claim we're trying to milk the Lorr treasury for our own profit," Zac retorted. "That's just not true. All we want is a fair deal, and funding for our new venture." He stopped short again. "And all I want is for my notebook to be returned."

"What makes this book so important to you?" I asked.

"It's…personal. As I said, I have my thoughts, my feelings in that book. And some of the experiments I conducted on certain strains of coal…"

"Coal?" I echoed. "Your delegation is dealing in coal?"

"That is one of the resources under negotiation, but I'm not directly connected with those discussions. I'm here to attend classes and lectures in organic chemistry at the Advanced Academy," he explained. "And to discuss several of my own findings with my colleagues from Lorr and Norland and South Coast. All my notes are in that book, so you see, I must have it, and soon!"

Merciful Founders Faith!. This character was a Boffin, one of those high-minded types who try to probe the mysteries of the innards of New Earth. Scientists, they call themselves. No wonder he was in a stew. One word of his indiscretions with a male licensee, and he'd be on the first transport back to Contramont. Goodbye to any hopes of advancement among the other Boffins, and whatever he'd been working on would be debunked as rotten at the source.

I shoved the form and the stylus closer toward him.

"Write down exactly what you want me to do, and pay me the silver," I told him. "Lorr coins. Conty credit chits are no good to me. I'm not about to go across the mountains to collect them."

"I have silver," Zac assured me, and laid out three coins. "You can contact me at the Strangers Hostel across Academy Way from the Advanced Academy in the Industrial Sector when you find the book." *When*, not *if*. At least he had that much confidence in me.

I nodded and added my signature to the document. "What does this thing look like?"

"It's about the size of my hand." He demonstrated. He had a fairly large paw for a Boffin. They tend to be scrawny types. "Plain paper between leather covers. Written by hand."

"Go back to your hostel," I told him. "I'll be in touch. As soon as I find your book, I'll send a message."

He started to say something, then thought better of it.

"May the Father and Son be with you," he said,

He left me wondering just what was going down with the Contramont Miners' Trade Delegation. Someone had laid out a lot of coin and effort to lure them into what they considered "sin", but to what end? What was so special about this new venture the Miners were pursuing? I made a mental note to find out.

I filed the form away in the bottom side drawer of my desk, then sat back and formulated a plan of attack.

Under normal circumstances, I'd get background on the client before I took on the case, but I had no sources for information on Contramont Boffins. My usual founts of information, my landlords Jake and Holly, were useless. As the leading couturiers in Lorr, they have their fingers on the pulse of Lorr society, but they don't know anything about Contys. The males all wear those cotton bibbed blue trou. The females? Who knows? Most of them aren't allowed to travel out of their mountain hideaways, and the very few that have been seen in Lorr weren't spending any coin on clothing.

Since this Boffin was a newcomer, I couldn't ask my contacts in Admin, either. Transients are supposed to register with the appropriate Guild, which forwards the information to Admin, but Boffin Zac wasn't connected with a Guild yet. Many Boffins affiliate with one or another of the Guilds, but only after they finish their studies and get certified in their specialty. Since Zac was still a student, he wasn't certified; and for all I knew, he'd head back to Contramont when he finished his courses.

I don't have any contacts at the Academy. I'd spent one very unhappy year there, fifteen years ago. I'd left suddenly for reasons I prefer not to recall, and I've never had much time for Boffins since. So, that line of inquiry was out.

If this venture of theirs was being sponsored by someone in the Banker's Guild, I might have asked one of *them* for an opinion of the Conrtramont Miners and their negotiations. But I'm not too welcome in the Bankers'

Guildhall these days, not after I'd exposed one of their leading families' involvement in a plot to introduce false coin into the Lorr economy. Once I gave testimony in a legal hearing, my face was known and marked. No chance of my getting straight answers there, not even from disgruntled office drones.

I decided to go down to Entertainment Row and start asking questions there. Just in case someone didn't care to answer, I pocketed the sigil from the Assassin's Guild, a token of appreciation from Master Assassin Fee M'Farr. I hoped I didn't have to use it. I prefer to keep my relationship with the Master Assassin private, as does he.

I also hooked my small bludgeon onto my belt. I didn't expect to use that, either, but you never can tell when someone might take offense; and it's always a good idea to be prepared for anything that might come along.

Then I decided to check the Newsposts, and find out just what this Contramont Miners' Trade Delegation was about; and why the Banker's Guild was being so iffy about lending them money.

And what made this particular young Boffin a target for seduction and theft of private property.

ii

I headed for the Newsposts to see what the pundits had to say about the Contramont Trade Delegation.

You'd think that a place like Lorr, where every contract is put on paper, would have a better way of spreading information than Posting it; but the Founders put their public notices on central pillars when they came

10

here, before the paper mills got started, and that's the way it's been ever since.

Six posts stand in a circle at key intersections and at the bridges across the river to Flatlands. Every Guild, plus Admin and the Dark Ones, sends runners with notices to be attached to the pillars at set times; and the public can thus be aware of important actions, sales of merchandise—whatever the Guilds, Admin, or Dark Ones think people should know about.

And then there's Post Six, where anyone can post anything at all.

My favorite Newspost is the one at the intersection of Clothier's Alley and the Grand Boulevard. I found the usual crowd in front of it, shouldered my way through, and checked the notices.

Post One has the International News, which is where I'd find what the Contramont Miners were up to. I scanned the notices while I tried to remember what I'd learned about Contramont in Basic Education.

According to my old schoolbooks, Contramont was started by some miners about a hundred years ago when the coal and iron mines on this side of the Mineral Mountains began to play out. They thought they could extract more out of the other side of the mountains, but to get there they had to go the long way around. The Mineral Mountains are really steep, mostly jagged peaks and crags, the only passes being the ones carved out by rivers at the bottom of deep gorges. Those rivers are full of rapids and waterfalls, so not navigable by anything larger than a small canoe with a daredevil paddling and carrying a few packs of animal hides to the markets on the other side.

To reach their goal, Contramont's settlers went past South Coast, through the Drogo Straits and north on the Inland Sea, then inland. Those early settlers were tough, according to the mag stories, battling giant lizards to get to the raw materials they wanted, and opening mines on the far side of the Mineral Mountains—hence the name *Contramont*. They found plenty of iron ore, coal, and other useful resources, all right; the problem was getting it back to where the raw material could be made into something else.

They chose to track to Port Chicago, and built steamers to carry the ore and coal to the refineries financed in Pangkot by the moneymen in Lorr.

At least, that's what I'd been told. How much was myth and legend, and how much was fact? Not my problem.

Whatever the history was, Contramont is one of those places where explorers and boffins from more civilized places go to find rarities. The people who live there? Total cloddies. The stock character in a farce is the Conty visitor to Lorr who talks with a twang and gets taken in by sharpers…and then turns their tricks around and gets back at them.

Post One didn't have much about the current discussions, except for a brief notice from the Banker's Guild that listed the Delrey Bank as backing a possible trade agreement with the Contramont Miners, with the addition: "Details of said agreement to be posted when signed, refer to notice on Post Three for more information."

Someone was being very cagey about exactly what was on the table. I thought this over as I scanned the other posts.

Post Two is Local—nothing dire at the moment, just the usual jousting among Guilds. Merchants insisting on selling what Craftsmen made, Craftsmen claiming they should be able to sell their own products. Transporteers fighting Seamen about access to the landing sites for the big ships docking in Flatlands. Grocers complaining about the Dark Ones imposing fines against products the Dark Ones claimed were tainted and therefore inedible. Everyone scratching for an advantage. That's the way it goes in Lorr.

Somewhere in the mix was a bulletin stating that the Flatlands Guards were now to be called the Flatlands Force, to distinguish them from the official Lorr City Guards. It didn't make much difference; they're still under the direction of the Honorable Guild of Forgers, Assassins, Thieves, and Swindlers. Set a thief to catch a thief? I hoped the Flatlanders felt safer with that lot protecting them. I wouldn't.

Post Three: Financial. I thought I'd better take a look at that one, too, just to check on the state of the Contramont Mines output. I elbowed a couple of females in light wool jackets and trou aside to search through the assorted notices of sales of goods and financial deals. I shivered in the rising breeze. It was getting windy; the autumn gales weren't far off, and my jacket wasn't that warm, but I wasn't ready to drag out the heavy leather coat yet..

Buried under a notice about a sale of lined winter jackets at Gueirenich's Boutique, I found what I was looking for. A brief note stated, "The Delrey Bank is considering backing the new mines in Contramont, but no decision has been reached. Certain differences between the parties concerning the terms of the loan are pending resolution."

Translation? Delrey was asking for more kickback than the Contys were willing to give, and the Miner's Trade Delegation couldn't go ahead without funding, so things were at a standstill until one or another party blinked. Zac had said he wasn't involved directly in these negotiations, but just suppose he'd heard something or seen something, and jotted it down in that journal. It might not sit well with the higher-ups. That was something I could look into.

My eye was caught by the notice next on the post. The New Earth Airship Line was heading into bankruptcy due to a lack of funding. Not surprising—the whole idea of running a fleet of airships from one settlement to another is absurd. Airships are best left to the daredevils of the Aerial Corps.

A few of the Upper Tier of Admin have private airships, but the cost of running one, the possibilities for disastrous crashes, and the horrendous cost of setting up a whole chain of stations along the coast of the North Continent makes the thing impractical. It would take a huge infusion of capital, and the cooperation of all the settlements just to get the scheme off the ground. Anyone who'd invested in it must be taking a bloodbath.

Then I remembered how much Selva and Devon Delrey had invested, and snickered. Between bad investments and dicey negotiations, things were not going well for the Delrey Bank.

Post Four is Entertainment, today touting a new farce opening at Theater One and a drama at Theater Two. I like a good farce; I'd check this one out when I had the chance. Drama? I get enough of that at work. I decided to skip that performance.

Post Five is Sports, not something I'm interested in. I take no delight in watching two people slugging it out, and I don't bet on who goes faster than whom, on two wheels or four. And watching people chase a ball around isn't appealing, either.

I waited patiently while various people came and went, riffling through the items on Post Six while I considered the Delrey connection with this affair.

Selva was out of the picture, shunted off to a faraway lodge where she could stew in her own juice. After her fiasco with the Pangkoti pirate captain Ishka Kunine fizzled, no one would even speak to her, let alone include her in any financial dealings. Bad enough for her to conspire with Pangkot, but to use her family connections to undermine the Lorr economy with false coins? That was the ultimate disgrace.

Devon Delrey? An amiable cipher, married into the Vikk merchant clan. He'd managed to charm his way back into his wife's circle, after a lot of groveling and promising never to stray again; but his role was as a figurehead, smiling at social functions.

That left two Delreys still active in the Delrey Banks —Vernor, the senior member of the clan, devious and secretive, and Gorgeous Gyorgi, the youngest Delrey, just out of the Academy and with a reputation for mischief.

Either of them might have decided to sponsor a party at a Pleasure Palace to entice the straight-arrow Contys into an indiscretion that could be used as leverage in negotiations.

Maybe I should check with Jake and Holly, I thought. If anyone knew what was going on in the Upper Tier, they did.

I finally got through the crowd to where I could flip through the various papers tacked or taped or nailed onto the post. Mostly gossip, of the "Who saw who where" kind, with no names mentioned for fear of lawsuits. I looked through the newer postings for something like "Found, one small book, will return for suitable reward."

Nothing of that kind was posted, but someone was indignant about the Contramont Miners Trade Delegation.

"Our friends from across the mountains should learn better manners! It is unseemly to rouse one's neighbors at an early hour in the morning with loud revelry best suited to the Academy Youth Services during the Solstice Break. Signed, Resident of Garden Sector."

So, that was where the Contramont Miners were being stashed, not in the usual Travelers' Lodgings between the Grand Boulevard and Entertainment Row? Either someone was renting a house, or they were staying with a Lorr resident. But Zac wasn't staying with them, not if he had a room at the Stranger's Hostel at the Advanced Academy.

Another interesting point, which I would follow up on. But not right now.

I checked the rest of Post Six for more about the incident, but no one else seemed to know or care what the rowdy Contys were up to.

I glanced up at the sky. Not sundown yet, but soon it would be dark. Time to check out Entertainment Row.

iii

I made my way towards the river, moseying along the Grand Boulevard where the Upper Tier does its shopping, past the foot of Arriver's Hill to the Flatlands Bridge, where Entertainment Row begins. As I strolled through the gathering crowd, I thought briefly about stopping at my digs on Foodie Alley, over Fletcher's Food Shoppe. It was getting chilly, and I could have used a change of jacket, maybe a quick bite at the shop, and a chance to check Ficus for new leaves.

I decided against it. I'm too well-known on Entertainment Row to pretend to be an office drone or Pangkoti refugee, so no reason to change clothes. I live there, I use the Entertainment Guild Baths, and many of the Entertainers and Licensees have come to me with their small problems. In return, they give me information. One hand washes the other, debt for debt.

As for Ficus, I didn't want to seem too anxious. It wouldn't do any good, and might even inhibit the sensitive plant. And it wasn't all that chilly, not yet.

I went past the entrance to the alley with only a glance upwards. Ficus was just visible in the window, not much more than a stem with a few leaves. I'd leave it alone, for now.

I sauntered past the two theaters, one on either side of Entertainment Row. The audience for the afternoon performance of the new farce was just letting out of Theater One. Theater Two wasn't open for business yet, but a signboard announced the new drama would be shown tomorrow.

I stopped by the corner where Moggy sat with his array of string and percussion instruments. He's a big male, no hair on top of his head but plenty below the chin, barrel-chested and long-limbed. His voice cuts through the constant chatter on Entertainment Row with a repertoire of new and old songs, some from the Ships, some he writes himself..

"Oyo, Moggy," I greeted him. "How's business?"

He shrugged and glanced at his open instrument case. I took the hint and dropped a couple of bits into it.

"That won't pay my rent," he complained.

"There's more for information," I told him. "What do you know about Contramonters?"

"They tip worse than you, Drach. And they don't appreciate good music."

"I heard some of them were on Entertainment Row last night."

Moggy grimaced. "I saw them. I even played 'Across the Water' for them, one of the old songs from the Settlement Times. One of them stopped to listen, but their keeper hustled them along."

"They weren't on their own?"

"They had a guide. A youngster decked out in a multicolor kilt and matching jacket." Moggy spat. "Pfeh! He made sure no one got away from the group."

"Really?" I added a half-silver to the case. "Must have been a rowdy bunch."

"Farmer boys, miners. Ship songs are lost on them —all they know is their own howlers; and they weren't interested in music, they were after females. The minder kept telling them to be patient, they'd find better company when they got to the party."

"That's for the info. Thanks."

And off I went, thinking hard. The Contramont Miners Trade Delegation had been led to the slaughter at a high-tier Pleasure House, which matched what Boffin Zac had told me. Nice to know the client wasn't lying.

I spotted a couple of Licensees lounging in front of the Grand Casino. One was a newcomer, a strapping brunette in a skintight red dress, hair caught back in a glittering net. The other, less spectacular but more welcome, was Velda, Basher Bob's popsy, a redhead. She wore a green gown that suggested more underneath than her friend's too-obvious garb.

"Oyo, Velda," I hailed her before she could pretend she didn't see me.

"Oyo, Pola." She turned and took a step away from me. She didn't get far in those super-high-heeled shoes.

"A word, Velda." I blocked her escape. "I need some help."

"The last time I helped you, I wound up with sundew stings up and down my legs and a ruined dress," she shot back. "You owe me, Pola."

What could I say? "You're right, I do," I admitted. "And I need your help again."

"What kind of help?" She gave me the stink-eye.

"Nothing dangerous. I just want to know whether you or your friend saw the Contramonters on Entertainment Row last night."

Before Velda had a chance to deny even being on Entertainment Row, the brunette in red spoke up.

"You mean that batch of bib-wearers? Straight from the Minerals? Sure did. You couldn't miss them. What a bunch of cloddies!"

"That bad," I said.

"You'd think they never saw a female before," Velda added. "Gawking at every Licensee they passed."

"I heard they were steered into one of the Licensed houses," I said. "You don't happen to know which one?"

"Pegeen's Pleasure Palace," the brunette sneered. "I saw them going in."

"Very upper-tier," I commented. "The Contramont Miners must be generous."

"Not with their own coin," the brunette groused. "The character in the kilt wouldn't let them even talk with me and Velda."

"Being hustled, were they?"

Velda leaned closer and spoke softly. "A very select party, made to order. Word went out two days ago` Pegeen was looking for talent of a particular kind, Clarisse here tried for a slot, but didn't make the cut."

"You don't say." Someone was going to a lot of trouble to give these Contys a good time.

"But Emil did," Clarisse sniped. "If I'd know that was the kind of party it was going to be, I never would have bothered."

"I never thought Pegeen would go for a male-male setup," Velda commented "Someone must have greased her wheels with gold, not just silver."

"Emil? A joyboy? At Pegeen's?" That definitely didn't add up. Pegeen's Pleasure Palace is one of the most discreet Licensed Houses in Lorr, but strictly male-female. Same-gender couplings are accepted in other houses, but not Pegeen's.

"Don't ask me why." Clarisse 's shrug nearly shifted her frontage loose from its moorings.

"I hear they were a frisky lot," I said. "Someone scolded them for being too rowdy on Post Six."

Clarisse sniffed. "All I know is, they went in on foot, they had their fun, they came out, and were taken home by hired pedi-shaws. I was just going back to my digs when they passed me. Couldn't mistake them, not with those crazy blue trou!"

"You didn't happen to notice a tall young male, fair hair, beginnings of a beard, among the survivors?"

She shook her head. "Couldn't tell one from another. They were all howling some Conty song, or maybe it was a hymn. Something about a bear and a mountain. They weren't in any condition for seconds, that's for sure."

"Interesting." I turned to go.

Velda caught my arm. "Why the interest in Contramonters?"

"I have a client who thinks he left something behind at the party. Thanks to you, I know where the party was. I'll pay the debt at Smokey Joe's tonight. See ya there!"

And off I went, before she got too curious.

iv

I cruised along Entertainment Row, passing various Entertainers on shift change as well as people going to and from the warehouses on the Waterfront. Licensees tend to work at night, but the casinos run full-time, no breaks, and rotate their shufflers and rakers.

The cletstands between the casinos were doing a healthy business as people stopped to get their fill before or after work; and street hawkers bawled come-ons for meat-pies and other small treats to tide the passers-by over until they could have a fuller meal at home or at a foodshop.

I stopped at one of the cletstands wedged between the casinos. I can't stand clet—to me it smells and tastes like wet socks—but I was starting to feel the wind's chill, and this place sold hot chai as well as clet, so I got a mug of that. The server was a hardbitten ex-Licensee with an eye for the passers-by and a mouth full of invective.

"Interesting crowd," I commented, shoving aside a female in a cotton skirt and scarf who reeked of fish, and

22

a male in leather trou and vest who sported the sigil of the Fatsos on the shoulder. "Looks like everyone's come to Lorr before the winter storms set in. Pangkoti, Norlanders. I hear there's even a delegation from Contramont in town."

"Contys? Sure thing. I saw them last night, marching along, gawking at the lights and the females like they'd never seen one. Probably hadn't, either!" She snickered.

"On their own?" I hinted. The chai wasn't bad, lightly spiced and not too sweet.

"Oh, there was some youngster with them, in some of those new duds. Showing their knees? What good's that? Unless it's to make it easier to get what's underneath!" The snicker became a guffaw. "Which, from the look of him, wasn't much."

"Small? Skinny?"

The server winked. "Nothing to be scared of, that's for sure." She handed the Fatso a cup of clet. I finished my chai and moved away.

I sensed someone behind me. I got a whiff of an expensive scent over the usual fish-laden air of the Waterfront and the mixture of clet and cooking oil from the foodstands. Definitely not a perfume the usual residents of either Fishmarket or Waterfront would wear. Maybe Upper Tier gone slumming?

I turned around, casually scanning the crowd, but I didn't see anyone who matched that scent. I didn't know if someone was following me, or just out for a stroll; but I'd remember that scent if I ever encountered it again.

My olfactory powers aren't as good as they are when Ficus is in full leaf. It was gradually recovering from its near-extinction, its stem hardening enough to carry a leaf or two; but even with applications of clet powder and bonemeal, it was struggling. I helped as much as I could, but plants have their own sense of time. At least, Ficus had given me a small spritz when I breathed on it that morning. Not much, but enough to give me a slight sensory edge on the rest of humanity.

I sauntered along, trying to catch a glimpse of my follower. Not easy in a street that was starting to fill up with mechs and techs heading to the bridge leading to their homes across the river in Flatlands. I thought I caught a flash of a gaudy pleated skirt as I turned the corner into the alley lit by a red lantern. No need for a signpost—those who wanted pleasure knew this was where to come for it.

Just a row of attached houses built in the old style —cinderblocks faced with brick, windows on either side of a wooden door, red-glass lantern over the door to signify what lay inside. No one knows why a red lantern —it's something from Old Earth, but there it is, and it hasn't changed since the Founders decided to make sex legally available for a fee as part of the Landing Operation's Rest and Recreation.

I scanned the row of blank-faced houses. One was Pegeen's, but which? I decided to trust to chance and knocked on the largest door, which was carved with a suggestive squiggle that could have been male and female organs intertwined.

A large male answered my knock. "We're closed."

"I'm not here for a futter," I told him. "I just want a word with the manager." I showed him the sigil from the Assassin's Guild.

"We don't want no trouble with the Fatsos," the doorkeeper assured me. He left the door open while he looked within for more instructions.

"There isn't any," I said, easing past him. "I just have a few questions, and I'll be on my way."

I was left in the front hall, a narrow space with a selection of interesting drawings on the walls, while the doorkeeper went up to the next floor in search of Pegeen.

She descended the stairs, a regal female about ten years older than me with pale hair swept into a high puff and classic features—oval face, straight nose, level brows. I immediately recognized the elegant trou-and-jacket ensemble as the most recent creation from Jake and Holly's. Clearly, a female of taste and refinement, not to mention coin.

She looked me over with a hard pale-blue gaze, and led me through the hall to her office. It might have been a match for mine, except the furnishings were a lot more comfortable, the desk was uncluttered, and the cabinet behind it held neatly stacked ledgers instead of scraps of paper.

"Pola Drach." She pronounced the name with a twist of the lips and an accent that tried to be Admin but wasn't quite. "What brings you here? If you're running an errand for Master Assassin M'Farr, you can tell him I run a clean house, according to the regs. I'm in good standing with the Entertainment Guild. And I am not going to knuckle under to the demands of rowdies, no matter whose sigils they carry." She glared at me. "They may *not* arrive unannounced, and I will *not* remove paying customers to accommodate them."

I'd heard some of the new Pangkoti recruits were getting out of hand, but now I had direct evidence. M'Farr may have bitten off more than he could chew when he took them into the Guild.

"I'm not here for Fee M'Farr," I explained. "I just used the sigil to get your attention. I'm here on behalf of a client who says he lost something in this house last night. He doesn't care how or when it's returned, he just wants it back. No questions asked, and he's willing to advance a reward," I added.

Pegeen's expression hardened. "I've told you, I run a clean house. There may be some people who abuse the trust of their patrons, but not here. I will not have thievery. I have told my staff, anything left behind or dropped in the course of events must be turned over to me immediately, to be returned to its owner."

"Very honest of you," I said.

"Just good business," she replied. "An establishment like this depends on its reputation for fair dealing. It's not worth losing over gewgaws and shinies!"

"The lost item wasn't a gewgaw. It was a book." I watched her face carefully.

"A book?" She looked totally blank. "I don't think any of my people found a book."

"It was left here last night," I repeated. "By one of the Contramonters."

She grimaced. "Oh, them!"

"Not your regular patrons?" I suggested.

"Certainly not!"

"A private party, then?"

She nodded. "Arranged by one of my most loyal patrons. "

"I heard you hired extra staff," I said. "Even joyboys. Not usual, from what I've heard about this house. The patron must be really generous."

"I do not usually hire outside help," Pegeen confirmed. "But the patron suggested one or two persons who would, ah, amuse his guests. And since he paid the bill, I could not refuse."

"I see."

And I did. Houses like Pegeen's Pleasure Palace depended on wealthy Upper Tier patrons for their survival, no matter what the regs said about equality. I knew better than to ask the identity of the mysterious patron. No matter—I'd find out sooner or later. Better sooner than later, but I'd find out.

"According to my client, he had intimate relations with a joyboy called Emil," I said. "What can you tell me about him?"

"Very little," she said through stiff lips. "The patron said he would send several young males around. He thought some of the guests from Contramont might desire a change of pace, as he put it. Emil was one of them. The patron swore he had been seen by a medico in the last week, and there was no reason to doubt him. I interviewed Emil myself. He was personable, not pushy, and quite polite. He was attractive, if you like them slender, dark, and sleek. I did not see him going upstairs, but presumably he did, since your client attests to his activities."

"And when the party dispersed?"

"He left. I do not know where he went. There was… some disturbance…when the Contramonters were escorted from my house."

"So I've heard," I muttered.

Pegeen's voice rose. "I have never had the Guards called! Never! I have already informed the patron. I will not have this kind of disturbance in my establishment. Bringing the Assassins to this place was bad enough, but inciting them to interact with paid patrons, and then summoning the Guards! I would never have taken the commission if I thought those people would react in that manner. Not for all the gold in Lorr! Drawing the Guards!" Her Flatlands accent overtook the fake-Admin in her agitation.

"Regarding Emil." I brought her back to the subject at hand. "How did you contact him?"

"He came here on his own. He claimed it was at the request of the patron."

"You must have some contact point for him, just in case you need him again." I smiled confidingly. "Not that you will, of course. But it's always a good idea to have the information."

Pegeen bit her lip. "I do not encourage male-male unions. However, as you say, just in case." She turned to one of the ledgers on the shelf behind her, opened it, and ran her finger down a page.

"If you think he has this book you're looking for, you might be able to find him at the Green Dragon Cafe, where most of the male Licensees gather. And I have been told there is a particular lodging-house on the border between Waterfront and Fishmarket, run by a female called Mama Gerda, which caters to the joyboys."

That was all I needed to know. I stood to go, then turned back. "One more thing. May I speak with your cleaners? One of them might have seen this book and tossed it away, thinking it was unimportant."

Pegeen's bland expression hardened into a frown. "My people know better than to throw away something they find in a room after a patron has left it."

"Still. Just to be sure?"

Pegeen thought it over, then said, "Come with me."

I followed her through the hall to the cleaners' quarters, a bleak room at the back of the house. There, three small brown females and a very young male sat on mats on the floor, ingesting something savory from bowls.

Pangkoti refugees. They aren't citizens, they aren't connected with any of the Guilds, and they take whatever work they can find for whatever someone is willing to pay them.

Pegeen announced, "This is Pola Drach. She wants to know if any of you have seen…" She looked towards me for more information.

"A book. Leatherbound papers," I added, in case these Pangkoti had never seen such a thing. "Left behind last night."

One of the females spoke for the group. "We clean rooms. We arrange bedding, we take damp sheets away. We do not take anything else."

"Did you see the joyboy, the one called Emil?" I asked.

The youngster started to say something in Pangkoti, but the female shushed him.

"Let him speak," Pegeen ordered. "If you saw something, you must tell me. You will not be punished," she added.

"And you *may* be rewarded," I said, producing a copper bit from my coin-pouch.

"I see Emil," the lad whispered. "He go away before Guards come."

"Did he, now?" Pegeen's eyes glittered. "I don't recall seeing him during the…the upset/"

"Could be it was he who called the Guards?" I hinted.

"If he did, I'll see to it he never gets another patron," Pegeen swore.

I handed the lad the copper bit, gave the women the Pangkoti blessing sign, and followed Pegeen back to the hallway.

"Thank you for your time," I told her "I am in your debt. If there's anything I can do for you…"

"You can inform Master Assassin Fee M'Farr that his people are overstepping their office, and there will be repercussions from the Entertainment Guild if they keep on the way they are going." Two pink spots that were not facepaint flared in her cheeks. "And when you see

30

Emil, tell him he will never work in my establishment again, no matter who the patron is."

"I will do that," I assured her, and headed back into the growing crowd on Entertainment Row.

I was certain none of the cleaners at Pegeen's had picked up that book. She wasn't lying when she said she'd never seen it and had no idea what it was about, or why it was important, and the servants didn't, either..

Emil was the key to this mess, and I set out to find him.

ν

I contemplated hiring a pedi-shaw to get me past the Waterfront to Fishmarket, then decided I might as well walk. It was sundown, end of the working day, and the warehouse mechs were heading toward the Waterfront Bridge and their little houses in Flatlands. The transporteers who run the carriers were changing shifts, adding to the confusion, one set coming from Flatlands, the other going the other way.

The fishing boats were pulling in, riding the tide that swelled the river. They docked alongside the piers, where eager hands grabbed the crates and baskets of still-flopping fish ready to be hauled away to the Fishmarket. Waves lapped at the pilings as the wind rose off the water, bringing the scents of fish and salt and mangrove trees…and expensive musky perfume. My follower was back.

I strolled along the docks, stopping a few times, making a show of catching a breath while I scanned the crowd

31

for that distinctive multicolor kilt and jacket among the undyed cotton trou of the sailors and the blue-dyed coveralls of the warehouse mechs. I spotted a few headcloths pushing through the crowd, heading south towards Fishmarket, like me. Pangkoti. The lucky ones, the ones who'd found work, maybe cleaning a warehouse, maybe helping the fishermen load their catch onto carts to be taken to the end of the pier, where the Dark Ones inspectors were waiting to process the catch. Once the fish had been pronounced edible, they would be sold to waiting customers.

The air here reeked of heated cooking-oil from food-shops where fish was fried, along with root-veg, ready to be taken home by the passing mechs, techs, and an occasional office drone from the warehouses. The crowd went both ways, some north to the bridge, some moving south to Fishmarket District and beyond it, to Industrial, where higher-tier techs mixed with lower-level boffins, close to the Advanced Academy.

I passed the long arcade that gave Fishmarket its name —a roof held up by stacks of old-style cinderblocks. Here the crowd became even more diverse, adding Pangkoti females in long skirts and draperies to the mix of males and females in standard Lorr gear.

The fishsellers bawling about their wares, the buyers haggling, the pteros squawking and swooping to grab a fish, and the yowling feral felines going after both fish and pteros hurt my auditory nerves. The odors assaulted my olfactories—fish, salt, vinegar and veg-sauce, frying oil, burning charcoal. I couldn't find the one following me, and decided to give it up for now.

A sharp whine penetrated the din. Everyone stopped what they were doing. Heads swiveled in the direction of the noise. I increased my pace, heading to the source of the siren. A City Guards skimmer was blasting away in front of a three-story house at the far end of the market. A Dark Ones skimmer hovered next to it.

A crowd had gathered, held back by a line of Guards, batons down, keeping the onlookers away from the house. I pushed forward to get a better look, only to be shoved back by the nearest Guard..

I felt a chill down my back as I recognized Captain Sara Atterson, top-tier, only called out on major crime scenes. Behind her, the gangling figure of Dark Kelvin, the Medical Examiner. Their presence meant only one thing—I was too late. Whatever Emil might have been able to tell me would never be told.

A pair of Dark Ones in the blue tunic and trou of med-techs carried something wrapped in a heavy cloth to their skimmer. A moan went up from the crowd, and a little old male in a yellow wraparound got past the Guards to peek under it.

"Emil!" he announced. In heavily accented Lorr Standard, he added, "Evil lives have evil ends." He followed that with a diatribe in Pangkoti. The men in headwraps and the women in skirts and bangles responded with loud cries of outrage. Everyone else looked away from the dreadful sight of Death.

I edged closer to the Guards skimmer.

"Stay back!" the Guard warned.

Atterson spotted me. "Drach? What are you doing here?"

"Eyeing," I replied. I looked at the squad. "I could ask the same of you, Captain. Since when does the City Guard get called out to Fishmarket?"

"Since Admin decided there needed to be a Special Squad to investigate things like this." She jerked her head toward the covered stretcher.

"I must have missed that," I said. "I've been eyeing in Flatlands."

She grimaced. "You should read Post Two more carefully. Admin set up the Special Squad, and I got the job four weeks ago, all as a consequence of your little stunt with Selva Delrey and her henchmen. Now I'm stuck following Fee M'Farr's new recruits. They're getting a little out of hand. "

I jerked my chin toward the body being stowed in the skimmer. "Is that a male called Emil? I wanted a word with him."

"On whose behalf?"

"You know I can't tell you that, Captain Atterson. All I can say is that this Emil might have had something a client wants."

"Oh?" Atterson's eyebrows went up. "A valuable something?"

"Only to the client," I said. "A personal journal. Not worth anything to anyone else. You didn't happen to see a small book in his quarters?"

Atterson's expression shifted from avarice to disinterest. "Not that I saw, but I wasn't looking for one. He didn't have anything like a book in his digs, not even a mag."

"How was it done?" I had to ask, ghoulish though it may be. No one in Lorr even likes to think of death, let alone mention it in public.

"Ask him." She gestured toward Dark Kelvin, supervising the bestowal. "All I know is the local Guard were summoned by the Mother's Guild female who runs the place. She went into Emil's room, saw him on the floor, and had the good sense to send for them. They took their time getting here. When they did, they took one look and called in the Specials."

"Be glad she did that much," I said. "Fishmarket's being run by Pangkoti rules these days." By their custom, males have free license to avenge what they consider wrongs on their own behalf. They're not about to pay the Fatsos to do what they can do themselves, and they never involve the Guards in anything if they can avoid it.

"Mama Gerda's not Pangkoti, she's a Norlander, and knows what's what," Atterson said. "But she didn't have much to say. Just that Emil was no bother, never made trouble, paid his rent on time. I guess the joyboy business must be looking up."

"Licensed sex worker," I corrected her. "

"Whatever." She shrugged. "My guess? A Sanctioned kill. Not anything for the Guards to worry about, as long as the contract was signed and paid for."

"What for?" It takes a while for a Death Contract to be filed, and a lot of coin as well. "What did Emil do to upset the Upper Tier?"

"Who knows? Maybe some patron didn't like the way he was treated. Maybe someone from outside Lorr

35

thought the joyboy might tell his spouse what he'd been up to in Lorr. If it's one of M'Farr's contracts, we can't do anything about it anyway—it's perfectly legal according to the regs."

True, but I still didn't like it. I had more questions than answers. Why turn the Fatsos loose on a joyboy? If it was a paid kill, who was paying? And what did any of this have to do with a missing book?

"There's one of the Fatsos in the crowd." I'd seen that particular big male a time or two. First at Smokey Joe's, with his trou at half-staff, then on Selva Delrey's boat. She'd called him Brutus. He was flashing a Fatso badge on the upper edge of his vest. He must have changed his employers and was now working for Fee M'Farr.

"Not my concern," Atterson said. "Let it go, Drach. Don't worry about Emil. He was just a joyboy."

"He was a human," I insisted. "And there aren't that many of us on this planet. Whatever he did for coin, he didn't deserve to end up like this. Besides, I've still got to find that book. If it turns up…"

"I'll let you know," Atterson said.

When lizards grow fur, I thought as the skimmer rose and sped away over the crowd, back to the safety of Guard Headquarters.

I strolled over to the Dark Ones' skimmer for a word or two with the med-techs who had carried Emil out. Instead, I got pulled aside by Dark Kelvin, his hair straggling down his back, his eyes sharp behind lenses, his long nose twitching, clearly irritated at being interrupted in his desire to get away from the scene.

"Independent Eye Drach," he hailed me. "Is this male one of your clients?"

"Not exactly. But I wanted to talk with him. When did this happen?"

"The Mother in charge found him this afternoon, around midday."

"And you're only investigating now?"

Kelvin sniffed. "It took some time before the Guards decided to notify the Administration, and for them to, in turn, notify Captain Atterson. I suspect this…" He waved at the body, now stowed safely in the skimmer. "…occurred near dawn this morning, either just before or just after."

"How?"

"A superficial examination revealed a sharp indentation in the flesh of his neck, the hyoid bone was broken, the thyroid severed. In my opinion, the weapon was a cord or wire, wielded with force."

"A garotte," I summed up. "Not used much in Lorr."

"Lorrans tend to go for the knife or bludgeon," Kelvin agreed. "I have heard some of the elite Assassins of Pangkot use this technique."

"It's a thought. Can I check his rooms now?"

"Are you suggesting my people cannot do a thorough search?" Kelvin's chin went up.

"They might not know what to look for." I lowered my voice to a confidential murmur. "I have a client who thinks he lost something, and that Emil might have found it and meant to hold it for ransom. If I could find it, it might shed some light on why Emil ended up… this way."

"My people are finished," Kelvin said, waving me away. "If you think you can do better, you have my permission to enter the scene." He joined his crew in the skimmer and took off, leaving me in the dust of the street.

vi

I stood there for a few moments, trying to think where to go next. My main lead was gone. I didn't want to go back to the client emptyhanded, but I wasn't sure if there was anything more I could do.

I heard a sniffle behind me. My hand on my bludgeon, I whirled around to face a young male, just over puberty, dark skin and hair, dressed in a multicolored kilt and Pangkoti red jacket.

"Was that...Emil?" His voice quavered.

"It was. You knew him?"

He nodded, too overcome at first to speak. "I served him. I helped him dress, and fetched his water. He was good to me."

"Was he, now?" I tried to sound neutral. It was the first sign I'd seen of someone truly unhappy at Emil's demise.

"He let me stay in his room when he was not there. He shared his food with me."

"And what did you do for him?"

The lad ducked his head. "I watched his belongings. I cleaned his clothes when he came from working. I did his errands, carried messages."

Bodyservant, I thought. "What's your name?"

"I am Jakki." He stared at the cinderblock house. "Where will I go without Emil?"

"You might ask the caretaker to let you stay and be her assistant," I suggested. "Why don't we go ask her together?"

I steered him across the street. A tall, fair female wearing a coarse striped apron with the Mothers' Guild sigil embroidered on the front over regulation heavy cotton shirt and trou stood in the doorway.

"Oyo," I greeted her. "How's business?"

She scowled at me. "You saw for yourself. One of the lodgers is done for. No one will take a room that's had…that…in it." She wouldn't say the evil words *dead one*.

"Why tell them?"

"It'll be all over Post Six. The landlord won't be pleased." She spied Jakki. "What's he doing here? I thought I told him to get out. I don't want him here."

"He's only a lad," I said. "And he's lost without Emil."

"I don't like his friends," the caretaker said. "They run around, make noise, steal from foodstands. Emil was polite, neat, paid his rent. The rest of the joyboy youngsters are rude, don't pay on time, blow weed, drink jack. I won't have that in this house. You ask anyone, they'll tell you. Mama Gerda runs a clean lodgings. The landlord won't have it any other way."

"They bring their work home with them?" I hinted.

Mama Gerda's lips tightened, and her expression grew grimmer, if possible. "They do not! What one does for coin, that is not my affair, but not in my presence, not in my house."

"What about this youngster?" I took another look at Jakki. Slender, almost scrawny, long nose, close-set eyes, tight-lipped mouth, dark complexion. Not especially pretty,, but he was afraid of something, for sure.

"He is a servant, and a spy. He works for the Fatsos."

"Only one," Jakki protested. "He saw me with Emil. He told me he'd give me coin if I told him who Emil saw and where he saw them."

"A spy!" The caretaker snorted. "Well, Spy Jakki, you can do your dirty work somewhere else. The lads are bad enough. I don't need grief from the Fatsos or the Specials. Find somewhere else to bed down!"

"Be kind." I tried to cajole her. "Let this lad stay in Emil's room for a while. You won't be able to rent it until the Dark Ones give the place a thorough scrub and the Pangkoti priest does whatever they do to keep ghosts and spirits away."

The caretaker thought it over. "Tonight, you stay. Once the place is cleaned, out you go!"

Jakki uttered something in Pangkoti that could have been a curse or a blessing and scampered up the stairs. I followed, eyes and ears open for anyone behind me.

Emil's lodging was a single room with a pallet-bed in one corner and a standing bed in the other. The one window was covered with a printed cloth. A small table held an alcohol lamp and a set of grooming tools—hairbrush, toothbrush, nail file, several small glass vials. I opened one of the vials. Mammal musk, very expensive stuff, imported from South Coast or Pangkot. A washstand with a jug and basin on top and a pail for the wastewater underneath was the only other furniture in the place.

A set of pegs on the wall held Emil's clothes—trou, shirts, jackets, all good quality. I checked the labels and raised my eyebrows. Emil had expensive tastes. Silk shirt, fine wool trou, nice beading on the jacket sleeves. Nothing shoddy, all hand stitched. From the Thieves' Market in Flatlands? Possibly, but not likely. I'd seen something like that jacket at the tailor's next to Jake and Holly's. Whoever was paying for Emil's services was very generous.

The floor was marred with a horrid splash of brown that made my nostrils quiver with the stink of excrement. He must have exuded it in his last spasms. It didn't add to the ambiance of the room.

I frowned at the standing bed. Not a particularly fine one—no headboard, just a flat mattress and one pillow. I reached under the mattress, shook the pillows, checked underneath, just to be sure. No book.

Jakki huddled on his pallet, his arms around his knees.

"What do I do now?" he moaned.

"If you have contacts with the Fatsos, you could enter the Assassins' Guild as an apprentice," I suggested. "Or you could register with the Servant's Guild."

"It takes coin. I have none." He held out a hand. "I could help *you*. You're Eye Drach, the one who finds things. You look for answers. I can help you find them.

41

I have friends, many friends, who go places and hear things."

I sized him up. He could be Eye material, but did I really want him?

"I'm looking for a book. Paper pages tied into a leather binding. About this big." I held out my hands. "The one who lost it thought Emil might have it. He's willing to pay coin to get it back."

"I do not know about a book." He didn't meet my eyes. He was lying. I tried again.

"You were here when Emil came home last night?" I persevered. "When was that?"

"It was late, nearly dawn. I was just waking. He sent me to the faucet downstairs to fetch water. When I came back, I saw him. He was on the floor. Then I was frightened. I did not want to stay where there was a death. I ran away to a Vikk-shop where I know someone who helps me sometimes. Then I heard the Guard skimmer, and I came back here, and saw them taking Emil out."

"Someone must have followed Emil home from Pegeen's," I mused aloud. "Someone killed him and took the book." I turned back to Jakki. "When you went to fetch the water, did you see anyone? Hear anything?"

"I thought I saw…something…on the stairs." Jakki blurted. "Big, black something! A djinn.!"

"Djinni don't exist," I told him. "What you saw was probably a big male. Maybe one of your Fatso friends?"

Jakki turned his head away. "I don't know. I didn't see a face. I can't tell anyone anything."

I left the lad sniveling on his pallet. I had enough information to come to a conclusion.

Fatso Brutus had been in the crowd. Fatso Brutus has a history of violence. A word with Fatso Brutus might finish this whole mess.

I headed back through the Waterfront to Smokey Joe's. It was as good a place as any to find him, as well as maybe some answers to the questions raised by Boffin Zac's notebook.

BRUTE FORCE

SMOKEY JOE'S IS THE PLACE WHERE THE UPPER TIER meets the Lower, where the riff and raff collide with the Better Half. It's one of the few wooden buildings left, built by the Founders back when trees were available in the hills surrounding what is now the City of Lorr. It's low and rambling, with wings and ells hidden behind its plain façade There are cellars under cellars, and it's rumored to have a tunnel with secret exits leading down to the river, built during the days when the merchant clans were warring with each other for dominance. That was back before the Guilds were established to settle matters quietly, without bloodshed.

It's not a fancy tourist attraction, with flashing electrics and noisy clings and clangs to attract attention. It's where local folks go for a quiet game of cards or dice, a mug of brew or a snort of jack, and a few minutes with a Licensee. It's also where people who don't want to be seen together meet for a quick confab.

It's the place where I go to get the gossip that doesn't penetrate the Upper Tier enclaves like Striver's Hill and Arriver's Hill. I can also get a brew and a bowl of whatever mixture of root-veg and meat the cook has concocted that day. It goes by the generic name of stew and usually tastes like sludge, but it's nutritious and only costs a few copper bits..

I waved to Sneaky Pete, the doorkeeper. He let me pass without checking my sigil or badge—I go there often enough so he knows who I am. He stopped a squad of sailors to check theirs, then waved another gang of mechs sporting Transport Guild sigils forward. He frowned away a noisy gang of youngsters in multicolored kilts. Troublemakers are not welcome in Smokey Joe's.

I stepped into the main room, willing my senses to dull down. The odors of old brew, fresh stew, and unwashed bodies assaulted my nasal passages. I let my eyes get used to the dim light and checked out the long bar.

Basher Bob, the big darkskin Independent Eye who helped me get started, was in his favorite spot at the end of the bar, with Velda next to him. He scanned the crowd for possible troublemakers or clients, or troublemakers who might become clients.

"Oyo, Basher, how's business?" I took the stool next to him and beckoned to Barkeep Joe. "One brew, and a bowl of whatever you've got today."I turned to Velda. "One for you, too?"

She shrugged. "I'd hoped for one of the top spots on Foodie Alley, but this will do. Did you find what you were looking for at Pegeen's?"

"Not exactly. I didn't find what the client is missing, but I found out who had it. Your joyboy friend Emil."

"No friend of mine," Velda sniffed. "He was a sneaky little twerp, always talking big, dropping hints of important patrons, but no names mentioned."

"He's not talking anymore. Someone took a cord to his throat." I accepted a mug of brew from Barkeep Joe.

"Any ideas who?" Basher Bob asked, too casually.

"The Special Squad is writing it off as a Sanctioned Kill, I saw Brutus in the crowd, probably checking out whether he was under suspicion."

Basher thought that over. "Sounds bogus to me. A joyboy? Not worth the coin for anyone to order a Sanctioned Kill."

"Captain Atterson is putting it down to the Assassins," I said. "Why not?"

"Because she's wrong, and so are you!" someone behind Basher boomed out. "I didn't do it! Tell her, Basher. I didn't do for Emil. Tell her!" He got louder and more insistent, drawing the attention of the drinkers at the bar.

I turned to see who it was. There hadn't been time for gossip to spread, so who knew?

It was Brutus. His bare arms bore a set of tattoos no Lorran male would even consider inflicting upon himself. What happens when tattoos cease to be fashionable?

"Easy," Basher soothed him, then turned to me. "Pola, we have to talk. What makes you think Brutus did it?"

"What's it to you?"

"He's asked for my help. Now, give, Pola. What makes you fix on Brutus?"

"I saw him in the crowd when Atterson's Specials took Emil away. If I spotted him, so did she. She's not blind, and she's not stupid. She's going to put two and two together…"

"And come after Brutus," Basher finished for me. But—"

"But I didn't do it." Brutus interrupted him. "I was there, sure, but I didn't do the job on Emil."

"And he wants me to find out who did," Basher said. "Before the Guards get the wrong man locked into a detention cell, and not even Fee M'Farr can get him out."

"Why drag me into it?" I asked.

"There are a few complications." Basher hesitated, then blurted out, "I'm not good with the Upper Tier, and Brutus says there may be a Delrey connection."

"Delrey?" I thought that over. "I'm not very popular with the Delreys right now. I don't know how I can help you if they're involved."

He didn't give up. "Pola, you owe me. Me and Velda got you out of a nasty spot not too long ago. It's not too much to ask for a little help with a client."

I did owe him. He'd helped me drag a very reluctant female out of Smokey Joe's, through the back of the place, getting stung by sundews in the process. He'd been out of commission for a week, and Velda was out a really spiffy dress.

"Let's find somewhere quiet, and you can tell me about it."

I looked around, spotted a table in a far corner, and led Basher, Brutus, and Velda to it. I beckoned a server, told him to bring my stew when it was ready, and prepared to listen.

"So, Brutus—Is that your real name?" I gave him a bland smile.

"It's what Banker Devon Delrey called me when I took service with him," he said, with a shrug. "I guess it's as good as any. My birth-name isn't for anyone not of the clan to know."

"Then Brutus it is. What's your story? What were you doing when I saw you in Fishmarket? Why were you in that crowd?"

"I live there. Not in the same house as the joyboys," he amended hastily. "The one across the road from it. Me and Casak and some of the others who got stranded here when Captain Kunine took off.

"He'd rented us out as bodyguards to Banker Devon Delrey, and Banker Devon passed us on to his sister, Banker Selva. After the Delray woman…" He stopped, remembering his manners. "That is, Banker Selva Delrey was taken away, Banker Vernor Delrey kept Casak on, sent him up to the mountains to keep an eye on her. He let the rest of us go, and said he couldn't afford to pay us. So, we found lodgings, and took work where we could."

I'd been responsible for getting Selva out of Lorr. I hadn't thought about her henchmen. Not too much work for hardbodies in Lorr these days.

"I heard the fellas talking about the Assassin's Guild," he went on. "How they were looking for recruits, folks who wouldn't mind working in Flatlands, part of something Master Assassin M'Farr cooked up. It sounded like a cushy job, so I signed on. It's not bad work, but kind of boring, watching warehouses and manufactories across the river. But it brings in the coin, and it's almost respectable."

He took a swig of brew. "I got a doss at a lodging-house in Fishmarket. There's plenty of Pangkoti there, food I can eat, even a puja—a temple to Mata Diva, al-most like home." He heaved a sigh. I never thought of those hardbodies as getting homesick for Pangkot, but even a hardbody is human.

The server emerged from the kitchen and deposit-ed a bowl of broth in front of each of us. Root-veg bits bobbed next to some kind of meat. I wasn't sure if it was fowl, reptile, or mammal, but it was protein, and I was hungry. I dug in while Brutus went on with his tale.

"Still, it's not a lot of coin comes with the job, so when there's a chance for a little extra, I don't turn it down."

"And what does the Guild have to say about that?" Meaning does Fee M'Farr allow his so-called Flatland Forces to take outside work?

"He don't know about it. I figure it's all right."

"Don't be too sure," I warned him. "Fee M'Farr likes to be on top of things. Just because he doesn't make a fuss about the extra work, it doesn't mean he doesn't know about it."

"Or doesn't mind, so long as the Guild gets its cut," Basher inserted. "Was the joyboy one of those extras?"

"I didn't do the joyboy," Brutus insisted. "I wasn't paid for that. All I was supposed to do was get the…the thing…"

"A book?" I guessed.

He stared at me. "How did you know? That's what the fella said I was supposed to get. He said it was stolen property, that Emil had taken it and this fella wanted it back. I was to go to Emil, get the book, and turn it over to the fella. He gave me coin, said I could keep whatever was left after I got the book."

"And you thought you'd just take the book and keep the coin?" I fished a piece of gristle out of the bowl.

"I knew Emil. I'd seen him coming and going from the house across from ours. He was one of those skinny sorts, not that tough. I figured I'd show him a blade, he'd cave, and I'd have the thing *and* the coin, and I'd hand the thing over to the fella, and that would be that. Easy coin. But someone else got there before me."

I took a sip of brew. You can never tell what Smokey Joe's brew will be like. This batch was better than most.

"This fella. The one with the coin. When and where did he give you this…assignment?"

"It was last night, after I checked in at the guardhouse by the Flatlands Bridge. I'm supposed to do that when I go off duty," Brutus explained. "Otherwise, I don't get paid.

"I have to sign in when I go over the bridge and sign out when I come back. This fella was waiting next to the guardhouse. He called me over, told me what he wanted me to do, and handed me the pouch with the coins."

"And you took them."

"I was going to report it to the Guild, after I finished the job and gave the fella his book." Brutus whined.

"Of course you were," I murmured.

"And it wasn't all that much, only eight silvers. No telling how much I'd have had left if I had to give some of it to Emil." Brutus looked from me to Basher, seeking approval.

Not that he'd do that. More likely grab the book and leave Emil bruised and bloody, but alive.

I took another bite of stew. "And just how were you supposed to get this book back to the fella?" The more I thought about this, the dicier it seemed.

"I was supposed to turn it in at the guardhouse, and he'd pick it up there."

"I see." And I did. This mysterious male probably had given the Guardsmen on duty a small token of esteem to hold the package for him until he came to pick it up. Not unusual in Lorr—City Guards were just as eager as the Flatlands Force to pick up a few extra coins here and there, and a favor for someone Upper Tier might lead to something bigger. "So, then what did you do?"

"I took the coin, and I went back to my doss," Brutus took up his tale. "It was late, it was dark, I was tired. I didn't see any hurry to get on with the chore.

"I figured I could get to Emil some time during the morning, after I had a snooze and it was light enough to see by. I'd go across the street, go up to his room. Once I cornered him, I'd get the book and take it to the guardhouse before I did my next shift. But like I said, someone else got to him. Not me!."

"So you say, but is there anyone who can vouch for you? Someone who saw you coming in at night? The caretaker or one of your hardbody pals? Anyone who can confirm that you didn't leave your room until after midday?"

Brutus frowned into his mug of brew. "They were all asleep when I got in, but someone was stirring when I got up. I don't know who, though."

I thought that over while I ate more stew. "So, what were you doing in the street when the Guards showed up?"

"I was in the joyboys' house," Brutus admitted. "I went in around midmorning, when Mama Gerda went down to the market getting the day's supplies. I climbed up the stairs. I didn't know which room was Emil's, but there was a door open, so I looked in. I saw the body and got out fast. There might be ghosts, and I don't want no part of them." Pangkoti may not mind saying the evil word, but they have a lot of superstitions about spirits.

"You saw the body," I said. "There was light in the room? A lantern?"

Brutus hesitated, glancing at Basher.

"Tell her," Basher ordered. "And don't bother to lie. She can smell it if you do."

At the moment, this wasn't as true as it was when Ficus was at full strength, but I could still detect changes in bodily aromas that indicated stress. Brutus was exuding stress, but I wasn't sure why.

"There was light from the window. Like I said, the door was open. I took a look, saw the body on the floor, and got out. Nothing else. I didn't even go into the room. I didn't step one foot near him!" His voice rose, drawing attention to our table.

Basher shushed him. "What then?"

"I wanted to go to my doss. Drink some jack, figure out what to do. I didn't want to think about what I'd seen. Then I heard a yell—Mama Gerda must have come back from her errands. I figured she'd seen the... what was there.

"The rest of the fellas in the lodgings went into the street to see what was going down, and I went with them. It would look queer if I didn't. Then the local guardsmen come, and they must have sent for the Specials and the Dark Ones. And that's that." He finished his story and looked from me to Basher and back to me. "And that's all I can tell you, because that's all I know."

"Basher, what do you make of this story?" I digested it with the stew.

"Brutus says he didn't do it," Basher said.

"And you believe him?"

"He's paid me three silvers to believe him."

"Good silver, or Pangkoti funny money?"

"Not funny, Pola. I'm inclined to agree with Brutus. He didn't do Emil."

"I saw him in the crowd at Emil's lodgings. Someone claims he saw someone a lot like him go into the house."

"You mean Jakki?" Brutus shrugged. "Could be he saw me in the house. I didn't see him, but he kind of lurks around, looking for a coin or two, him and his street-lizard pals. That still don't mean I did the deed, and I tell you, I didn't."

"Any ideas who did?" I scraped the bowl to get the dregs of the stew. It wasn't bad—a little heavy on the salt, but the meat was reasonably fresh and the root-veg crunchy.

"Not me." Brutus shrugged. "Could be almost anyone. That Emil was a piece of work.

"Not that I have anything against joyboys—everyone's got to make a living—but there are some that just set my teeth on edge, and he was one of them. Too slick by half. Sashaying here and there, pretending to be grand, putting it on about his Upper Tier connections, wearing the fanciest duds, giving coin to Mata Diva's puja. Coming to chant and pray there. All for show, not because he really believed."

"Upper Tier?" I echoed. "Any names named?" Male-male pairing isn't all that daring, but not something to boast about, either. From the point of view of population growth, a little futile, but if that's your taste, no one in Lorr is going to make a fuss about it. On the other hand, hiring joyboys? Comes under the same heading as taking popsies off the street—just not done by the Admin Uppers or the top-tier Guildmasters who imitate them.

"He never said who. Just flashed his duds, hinted that he'd have more and better, made a big showing at puja."

"What else can you tell me about this mystery male… it *was* a male? The one who called to you when you got over the bridge? The one who gave you the coin?" I got back to Brutus's first story. "What did he look like? Sound like? Big, small, fat, thin, tall, short?"

"It was dark. I finished my shift just after moondown, and the electrics go off about then. But, yeah, I'd say it

54

was a male. He was tall, not fat, wrapped in some kind of cape or blanket."

"Hat?"

"Maybe. Something on his head, anyways. And a low voice."

"How did he sound? Did he speak Lorran, or something else?"

Brutus looked down, realized there was food in front of him, and began spooning it into his mouth as if he hadn't had a square meal in days.

"Lorran, but different from what they talk in Fishmarket or Flatlands. He sounded...I don't know how to say it...like he had something wrong with his nose? And he used big, fancy words. He said..." Brutus closed his eyes, trying to picture the scene. He put on an Admin's drawling accent. 'An object has been purloined. The Licensee Emil has taken what is rightfully mine. You will find it and return it here.'

"And then he gave me the pouch. It jingled like it had lots of coin, but it was just silver and copper bits." Brutus reflected a bit more. "I thought I'd heard him before, but maybe not. All those high-toned Uppers sound alike."

This didn't make sense. I did a mental time-check. If the book had been taken during the whoop-de-do at Pegeen's, how did this character even know it was missing? Unless Friend Boffin Zac had been set up...

A commotion across the room interrupted my musing. Boots clumping, chairs being shoved, people yelling.

"Oh, Death and Destruction!" Basher swore. "Look what just walked in!"

I turned to take in the party that had just burst into Smokey Joe's.

Three young males in the multicolored jackets and kilts that marked the most fashionable of the Admin lads swaggered across the room, along with two more in tight trou and silk shirts.(joyboys, I guessed—street licenses, not house staff), and another young male in the blue trou and straw hat common to Contramont. They commandeered the table immediately in front of the small stage. What was Boffin Zac doing with this rowdy lot?

Behind them loomed two hulking Pangkoti bodyguards in black leather vests and trou, arms bared to show tattoos.

"It's Gorgeous Gyorgi Delrey, as I live and breathe," I said to Basher. "And he's brought some friends along for the ride. How'd he get past Sneaky Pete?"

"Probably paid his way in," Basher snarled. "And what's that piece of fluff doing here?"

Hovering a few steps behind the youngsters was someone I never thought to see in Smokey Joe's—Reg Bonwit. He's the eyes and ears of Julian Hunt, better known as The Brain.

Hunt never leaves her house on Arriver's Hill, and sends Reg out to collect information; but Reg Bonwit doesn't come anywhere near Smokey Joe's. He's more likely to be seen in the big casinos, romancing the Admin debs or the Merchant's Guild clan females. Whatever he was up to, it had to be business, and since The Brain wasn't interested in any but the Upper Tier, that meant he was most likely there because of Gorgeous Gyorgi.

This was not going to be the usual night of casual companionship at Smokey Joe's. I sipped more brew and waited for developments, one eye on the table with the Admin lads. Things were about to get very interesting, and I wanted to be ready for whatever happened.

iii

Reg glanced around the room, spotted me and Basher, and slithered over to our table. He's a snappy-looking male about my age—pale skin, brown hair and eyes, straight nose. Hair neatly cut, black trou-and-jacket set from one of the better tailors in Clothier's Alley. My nostrils tingled at the whiff of expensive scent, musky and woodsy, definitely a Norland import, enough to cut through the miasma that permeated Smokey Joe's. Not the exact scent I'd caught at Fishmarket, but close to it.

Basher growled something unpleasant and tried not to notice we had another male taking a seat at the table. Velda smirked. I wasn't so standoffish.

"Oyo, Reg," I greeted him. "How's business? What brings you to the dark side of the Row? Slumming?"

"Eyeing," he admitted. "Brain business."

He directed his gaze toward the table where Gorgeous Gyorgi and his comrades were making themselves obnoxious.

"I've been asked to keep an eye on that youngster." He nodded toward them. Gorgeous Gyorgi's better-dressed buddies were the heirs of the Construction and Transport Guildmasters, just out of the Advanced Academy and not yet settled into their respective slots in the Guildhalls. I didn't know the joyboys by sight, but their profession was pretty obvious. The odd one out was Boffin Zac, staring at the mechs and sailors at the other tables. They belonged at Smokey Joe's, but he didn't for sure.

"Which one?" I looked them over. Transport and Construction were yelling for service. Gorgeous Gyorgi was smirking at the lowlifes around him. The two joyboys were nervously tittering at something Gorgeous Gyorgi'd said.

And Zac? He just looked around, red-faced with embarrassment, not knowing how to behave in this company.

"That would be telling." Reg smirked. "The Brain has a client who wants information, and I've trailed this lot to get it."

"And you wound up here?"

"Gorgeous Gyorgi Delrey decided to come check out the place. To hear him tell it, his big brother Devon said it was vile, so of course he had to see for himself," Reg said with a grimace. "How's the refreshment here? "

"The brew's drinkable today. Ask Basher about the jack, I never touch the stuff." I had, once, and that was enough for me.

We retreated to the far end of the bar as a pair of buskers took the stage. Manager Joe, whose real name no one knows, since every server in the place is called Joe, joined them and yelled for quiet.

"Thanks to a special patron, we have a great treat for you," he announced. "Give your attention to Randi and Kira!"

This was a step up for street musicians, and I had to wonder just who was the generous soul who had paid the extra Entertainment Guild fee to move them indoors. Busking isn't a steady profession, and Randi and Kira are good, but not that good.

They broke into song, a ballad about a ship's crew wrecking a port while on shore leave. It had salacious verses and an infectious chorus that everyone joined in on by the third repetition.

Basher didn't sing. He kept his eyes on Reg, who watched Gorgeous Gyorgi and his crew. I left the bar and joined the crowd that had followed Randi and Kira into the place, edging through to a spot just behind Gyorgi's table..

The song ended, to great applause, and people threw coins onto the stage. Randi bowed. Kira looked at the coins, unsure whether to pick them up herself or wait for one of the servers to do it. They'd be shared with the Entertainer's Guild eventually, no matter who picked them up.

"And now, a new song for some of our friends from Pangkot," Randi announced. He started a martial ditty about a group of soldiers on campaign. It seemed to have some meaning for a pack of hardbodies at the other end of the bar. They started to grumble as the song progressed.

I maneuvered myself just behind Zac's chair. Bending over, I murmured "If you aren't happy, get out now, while Delrey isn't looking."

He nearly jumped out of those bibbed trou as he hopped out of his chair.

"Independent Eye Drach! What are you doing here? Are you following me?"

I pulled him aside, away from the others.

"I came here to eat dinner. And I could ask the same of you. This place isn't on the tourist circuit, and Academy students have their own gathering places. What brings you to Smokey Joe's?"

"I was invited to join the party," he said. "Junior Banker Delrey came to the Stranger's Hostel, asking how I was feeling after our excursion yesterday. He said he and some of his friends were going to dinner, and they would be pleased if I joined them.

"I wasn't sure I wanted any more of that company, but I remembered Elder Mackintosh thought I should accept Junior Banker Delrey's invitations whenever he asked. Master Banker Vernor Delrey is one of those with whom the Trade Delegation is dealing, and Elder Mackintosh said I should cooperate with him in keeping the Delrey clan happy.

"He suggested I accompany Junior Banker Delrey to…to wherever he wants to go," Zac ended lamely. "I'm not used to this sort of place. They drink alcohol here!"

"Then make your excuses and get out," I said. "Tell them…something. Say you've got to be up early for classes. Or that you have a lecture to give."

"I can't lecture without my notebook!" Zac hissed at me. "Have you found it? Did you find Emil? Did he have it?"

"Emil isn't saying much to anyone." I turned Zac towards the door. "We have to talk. Let's get out of here."

The singers were attracting more attention than they had bargained for from the hardbodies at the other end of the bar. They weren't joining in the choruses. They were actively protesting the verses.

Randi got to the point of the song. "There's no such thing as an honorable death." was the final line.

The hardbodies stood up, ready to disagree with him.

Gorgeous Gyorgi applauded the singers, then looked around and realized one of his followers had left the table.

"Zac!" No title, no honorific, not even *Boffin* or *Student*. "Come over here!" he yelled, as if he expected to be obeyed.

Zac looked from Gyorgi to me and back to Gyorgi.

"I think Friend Garber has decided to leave," I said over my shoulder, pushing Zac farther away from his so-called friends..

"You're Pola Drach. The one who got my sister banned from Lorr." Gyorgi stood up and waved an accusing finger at me.

"She deserved it," I countered. "She conspired with an enemy of Lorr to subvert the currency. That's a mine-stint offense. She got off easy."

"It was no concern of yours," Gyorgi sneered. "You're just an Independent Eye. No Guild will have you."

It was the other way around. I've had offers, but I prefer not to affiliate with a Guild or the Administration. I stay Independent. That's my choice, no business of his.

"That's as it may be," I said.

I could sense someone behind me and got another whiff of expensive scent. Reg had left the bar to join me.

"Can I help here?"

"I think I can do this myself." I didn't want Reg involved in my business. Julian Hunt's boy wonder wasn't mine.

While I was maneuvering Zac away from the table, the hardbodies were starting to converge on the stage.

"Is this twerp bothering you, Pola?" Basher and Velda appeared behind Reg.

"Not really. One of Junior Banker Delrey's friends has another appointment and wants to leave," I said. "I thought I'd help this youngster find his way back to the Stranger's Hostel at the Academy. It's a ways across town, and he might get lost finding it. Friend Brutus?"

Brutus looked baffled. "You mean me?"

"I've got a chore for you. Come with us, and help us with this lad."

"What do you want me to do?"

"Just keep an eye on the lad while he's on the carrier."

Reg grabbed Zac by his free arm before I could stop him.

"You can take the carrier back," he told Brutus. "If you need more, this will get you a pedi-shaw back to your lodgings." He added a silver as an inducement.

Basher put in his two copper's worth with Brutus. "It won't take long, you'll be back here before you know it. And you'll have these two in your debt."

"Yes, but..." Brutus glanced at his countrymen, who were yelling at Randi. Manager Joe had summoned his own hardbodies, a brace of bearded Norlanders who

62

had no love for Pangkotis. Ethnic insults were being slung on both sides of the fight.

"Take care of the youngster," Basher urged him.

Gyorgi, backed by the bulkier Transport and Construction heirs, two Pangkoti hardbodies, and the skinny joyboys, announced, "This place isn't as amusing as Devon told me it was. I am leaving." He headed for the door.

Manager Joe stopped him. "There's a bill to pay. Jack and brew, and what you advanced for the music."

"Send the tab to the Delrey Bank." Gyorgi thrust Manager Joe out of his way.

"You'll pay it now!" Basher stepped forward.

"What's it to you?" Transport heir demanded.

"I work here," Basher stated, which he did, sort of. Manager Joe gave him free jack and food as long as Basher kept the hardbodies in line. Except right now, said hardbodies weren't paying much attention to Basher. They wanted to take a piece of Randi's hide for insulting their compatriots, implying their previous life-style wasn't all that noble.

A pair of Fatsos came out of the crowd.

"Brutus, these characters bothering you?"

Pangkoti hardbody Number Two stepped up to back Number One, getting into the path of a Fatso. The Fatso shoved Pangkoti Number Two. Number Two responded with a shove of his own.

And the fight was on!

iv

As bar brawls go, it wasn't particularly epic. I've seen worse, even been in a few. This one was more memorable for who was involved than how many punches were thrown.

I stepped out of the way when the Norlanders, Fatsos, and Pangkoti bodyguards went at it, dragging Zac with me. He shook me off and squawked in protest.

"I'm not a coward! I can fight as well as anyone else!"

"Sure you can, but this isn't your fight, and your Contramonter Elders wouldn't like you getting banged up in some brannigan," I assured him. "Let's get out of here, before the Guards come to break this up."

I looked around for support. Basher was slugging it out with the Pangkotis, who were after Randi, who was trying to protect Kira, who was snatching as many coins as she could from the floor of the stage. The Norlanders were just whaling away at anyone they could reach. Manager Joe was screeching something, but no one was listening.

I got hold of Zac again, Reg grabbed Zac's free arm, and the two of us dragged him towards the door. I dodged an infuriated sailor, whose mug of brew had been upended into his face by a man who'd fallen across his lap. The sailor yelled something rude in a South Coast dialect and shoved the hardbody off. Said hardbody shoved back, triggering another battle.

I unhooked the bludgeon from my belt and used it to jab the battlers out of our way . Between us, Reg and I maneuvered Zac around knots of fighters on our way to the door. Velda and Basher yanked Brutus out of the fray, and joined me and Reg, pushing Zac from the rear as we made our way through the crowd.

I had to use my bludgeon on a few heads, and Velda kicked at least one participant in the knee to make a path for us; but we got Zac and Brutus outside just as a squad of City Guards arrived.

"There's a fight inside," I told the largest Guardsman.

"Disturbing the peace is an offense!" he declared, and in they went.

We sorted ourselves out in the street by the light of the swinging electric lamp at the carrier station across the road from Smokey Joe's. The next carrier had just pulled into the terminus, disgorging the few passengers making their way back along the Waterfront to Fishmarket. The carrier line ends at the Waterfront; from there on, you're on your own, either via foot, two-wheel, or pedi-shaw.

Reg smoothed his hair, which had gotten ruffled in the fight. Velda arranged her dress, which had also been mussed and was sliding down her front, proving without a doubt she was female. Basher looked longingly after the Guards, but stayed with us.

I re-hooked my bludgeon onto my belt and twitched my jacket into place. Then, I faced my client.

"Allright, Friend Boffin Zac," I said sternly. "Where have you been since you left my office?"

Zac gulped and looked from one face to another. Basher, Reg, and I were waiting for an answer.

"I…I went back to the Academy, like you told me to. What's wrong? Where is my journal, and where is Emil?"

"Emil is dead," I said, brutally.

Zac gasped and went pale. "He...he can't be. He was well when I left him..."

"I told you. He's dead. Someone took a cord to his throat."

"Horrible!" He looked ready to faint.

"So, I ask again, what did you do between the time you left him and the time you got here?"

"You think...me? You think I...?"

"It was a possibility, but no, I don't," I assured him. "But you're my client, and I have to be sure you don't wind up the same way. That book of yours has got someone really upset, and until I find it, you won't be safe."

I turned to Brutus. "This youngster has to get back where he belongs. Take the carrier, get him back to the Strangers' Hostel at the Academy. It's in Industrial Sector, the carrier goes right to it. Make sure he goes inside. They'll take care of him once he gets there."

Zac started to protest. "I am not a child. I can take myself to the hostel. And you haven't found my book yet."

I was really getting tired of this youngster's whining.

"One brawl's enough for one night, Friend Zac. We have a saying in Lorr—you don't keep a feline and catch lizards yourself. I'm still Eyeing for you. which means you're paying me for my work. That includes my advice, which is for you to get back to the hostel and let me do what you're paying me for.

"I have a good idea where your book is. I can get it back to you by moonrise tomorrow. Come and see me at my office then."

I shoved Brutus and Zac toward the carrier. The Transporteer was ringing the bell, alerting possible passengers it was about to depart.

Brutus and Zac mounted the steps and sat on the benches. I could see their heads as the carrier moved forward. There was always the possibility one or the other would get off before they made it to the Academy, but I didn't think that was likely. Neither Zac nor Brutus was familiar with Lorr, and the electrics were starting to blink out on schedule, leaving the streets in shadow.

Both the gold and the silver moon were in crescent phase, so not much light from them. No point in walking dark streets alone when you didn't know where you were going.

I turned to Velda. "Have you had enough excitement, or are you heading back inside?"

She grinned at her companion. "Basher needed a good workout, but I think he's done for the night. I'll take care of him. You go home, Pola, and take care of your pet plant."

That sounded like the best idea I'd heard all day, but I couldn't do it. Not yet. I'd just remembered the one place I hadn't searched when I was in Emil's room.

I started the long walk down the Waterfront.

v

I wasn't happy about going back to Fishmarket. The Lorr City Council doesn't see any point in paying for electrics in a district that doesn't return much by way of tolls or rents—hence the steady blackout of the lamps. In their viewpoint, the folks in Fishmarket can stay home after dark or find their way with lanterns.

To that end, each house is supposed to have a lantern at the door, but they don't give much light, and householders put them out when they go to bed. No one in Lorr wants to risk fire, not in our high-oxygen atmosphere.

During the early Age of Settlement, there were really bad fires. After a while, no one built anything of wood, only cinderblock and brick. Smokey Joe's only survives because it's so close to the river, it's practically fireproof.

I looked up and down the street. To my right beckoned the lights of Entertainment Row, with my digs at the far end. To my left, the dark Waterfront, and darker Fishmarket.

I gritted my teeth and started walking along the pier. I could see my way only by the lanterns hung on the bows of the boats bobbing at their moorings and the two electrics at either end of the market building.

Behind me, I heard footsteps and smelled expensive scent. I whirled around, bludgeon in hand, to face Reg Bonwit.

"Easy!" He threw up a hand. "Not an enemy, Pola Drach! Just looking out for a fellow Eye."

"Looking for something someone lost?" I guessed.

"Or something someone wants found," he countered. "Hunt's client wants to know where certain funds went. So far, everything points to the Delrey Bank, but that's where the trail goes cold."

"Delrey Bank's been involved with a lot of dicey business."

"Including the Contramont Mines?"

I gave that some thought as we strolled along. I tried to make out more sounds and smells, but Ficus's gift was wearing off. The wind rose off the water, sending weird sounds through the openings in the fishmarket roof, and the stench of rotting fish and waterweeds overwhelmed almost everything else. Something was sloshing along the riverbanks, possibly reptiles hunting amphibians, possibly just the tide coming and going.

I nearly missed the subtle *whoosh* behind me. Reg didn't, and shoved me out of the way as a small stone clicked against the market wall.

Footsteps echoed off the wooden pier as someone ran away into the rising mist.

Reg had grabbed my arm before I hit the ground.

"Was that for you or for me?" I took a deep breath, and only got another whiff of his scent. Musky, expensive, but not the same as I'd smelled on my first trip down the Waterfront.

"Whoever it was doesn't want either of us to go on," Reg said, with a shrug. "They may be right. Like your friend Basher, one fight per might is my limit."

"Besides, the Brain won't like it if you get taken out," I sniped.

Reg stiffened. His relationship with the Brain is something no one really understands, least of all me.

"I think we'd better go back," I decided. "I can always go to Fishmarket when it's light."

"I saw a pedi-shaw at the carrier terminus. I can drop you off on my way to Arriver's Hill."

It was an offer I could refuse, but I didn't. He was right about one thing—one fight per night was more than enough. I wanted to think things over, and I couldn't do it on the Waterfront.

I let him pay for the pedi-shaw, and hopped out at Foodie Alley. My digs are in the middle of the row, over Fletcher's Food Shoppe, and I wanted something to take the taste of Smokey Joe's stew out of my mouth. A dish of sweet grain mush or a pastry would be a fitting end to a frustrating evening.

Ficus was waiting for me when I came up the stairs with my sweet, a mug of hot chai, and a jug of water for my morning ablutions. I had half my berry tart and chai while I checked my plant for insects.

Autumn is swarming season, and you never can tell what sort of creepy-crawly might decide to roost on a likely leaf. I gave Ficus a spritz of mineral water and a measure of bonemeal, finished off with a smaller measure of the powdered clet that had proved disastrous as a drink but great for stimulating plant growth. Then I moved its pot from the windowsill where I had placed it during the day to the small table where I write my notes.

"None of this makes sense," I told Ficus, stroking one of its leaves. "Young Boffin Zac gets lured into Pegeen's Pleasure Palace, he has sex with Emil, then he's hustled out so fast he leaves his notebook behind. And before he even knows it's gone, someone pays Brutus to get it from Emil, who may or may not know what it is, or why it is so important. How many people are after this thing? And what's in it that everyone wants?"

I had no answers to any of these questions. They would have to wait until morning.

I've since gone over and over what I should have done. Would it have made a difference if *I* had taken Zac across Lorr instead of Brutus? Could I have prevented a life from being taken?

At the time, it seemed like I had done the right thing, the sensible thing. By the time I found out I hadn't, it was too late.

BOOK-TRACKING

UP AT SUNRISE, I WENT THROUGH MY MORNING ROU- tine while I mentally laid out my schedule for the day —wash the face and other bits, arrange hair, and pick out an inconspicuous outfit least likely to draw attention on the street. Serviceable brown trou, white shirt, and my new heavy brown jacket that could be turned inside out to reveal a checkered lining.

I talked to Ficus as I brewed my morning chai and munched the remains of the berry pie for my morning meal.

"I've got to get to Fishmarket, check out Emil's digs, and find that book," I told it. "It's got to be somewhere. It wasn't in his bedding, but it might still be hidden in some secret hidey-hole I didn't see before. Or maybe in Jakki's pallet? What do you think?"

Ficus rustled its few leaves.

"Jakki has it? Could be, but why didn't he just give it to me when I saw him last night?"

Ficus didn't have an answer to that one.

"And I want to check out Brutus, see what his pals have to say about him. He was tied into Ishka Kunine, then the Delreys, now he's working with the Fatsos. Not a stable person, chopping and changing to suit the circumstances. And that story about being called to from the shadows? Sounds bogus to me."

Another rustle from Ficus.

"You're right, I won't find any answers sitting here drinking chai. I'll get over to Fishmarket, find out what I can about Brutus. And then I just might mosey over to Industrial and ask the boffins at the Academy about Zac and his notebook. "

I set Ficus in the window where it would get light. I gave it another breath to encourage it to put out a few more leaves, and it gave me a small dose of the pheromones that enhance my olfactory and auditory nerves slightly—enough to give me an edge, let me know who or what is sneaking up on me.

I draped a long scarf around my neck, tucked my coin-purse into a jacket pocket, hung the small bludgeon on my belt, and I was ready to face whatever was waiting for me in the streets of Lorr.

I descended to Entertainment Row. There was a nip in the air, a hint of winter on the way. I decided to splurge on a pedi-shaw and save myself the effort of braving the crowds coming over the bridge from Flatlands. Mechs, heading back to the docks and the workshops that hid behind the fishmarket, office drones on their way to their desks in the Business Sector, sales clerks going to shops on the Grand Boulevard. All either on foot or on two-wheels, all striding or riding to their occupations. No skimmers in Flatlands. That's for the Upper Tier.

We pedaled past the Flatlands Bridge and continued along the Waterfront. The fishing boats had already caught the outgoing tide, heading downriver, riding the current out to the estuary and the open sea beyond. The scows and barges from upriver moved into their places at the docks, offloading crates and baskets of vegetables and casks of grains.

Pteros and felines prowled, looking for whatever scraps had been left by the previous day's catch. Small lizards scrabbled in odd corners, trying to evade both species of predators while catching their own meals of creepy-crawlies.

I let the pedi-shaw driver do the hard work while I leaned back and enjoyed the sights and sounds and smells of the morning.

As we approached the line where the Waterfront District becomes Fishmarket, the aroma of incense increased. I could hear the *ting-ting-ting* of bells and the *jingle-jingle-thump* of a tambourine.

We pulled up in front of the joyboys' digs. A squad of Pangkotis in yellow draperies stood in the street, waving incense sticks and intoning prayers to a bell-and-drum accompaniment. I paid off the driver, who bowed reverently toward the musicians and headed back to the docks.

I assessed the crowd gathered around the musicians. Some might be mourning Emil, but I suspected more were just drawn to the music and incense, anything to break the slog of earning a living. I wrapped the scarf around my head in a gesture of respect and circled the crowd to the door. There Mama Gerda stood, broom in hand, sourly observing the scene.

"Oyo," I greeted her. "How's business? Who sent for this lot?"

She grimaced at the mourners. "They started before dawn this morning. The head priest says it's to keep the evil spirits away until Emil's soul finds peace."

"That's going to take a while," I said. "Maybe I can help ease their minds."

A second gang of Pangkotis, in red trou and jackets, heads topped with red felt caps decorated with tassels, joined the first. They added a wailing flute to the din, drawing more people to the scene.

"Emil must have been popular," I commented. "His passing is being remembered."

"Emil was a blowhard." Mama Gerda snorted. "When he had coin, he spent it. Where he got it, no one cared. As for them…" She nodded toward the musical combatants. "…they're from the two temples down the street. The yellow ones are for Mata Diva, the red ones are for Buda-Ganesha. Both are claiming Emil as their own. He gave to both of them."

"Have the Dark Ones released Emil's room?" I asked.

"It's been cleaned," she replied. "Once those priests finish, I can rent it again. It won't be easy, not when people know what…what happened there."

"There are new people coming in all the time. They won't know about Emil," I pointed out. "The other joyboys are still around. And what about that youngster, Jakki?"

"He's gone." Mama Gerda sniffed. "Lit out early, before sunup, just before those priests arrived. Good riddance, him and his street-lizard friends. They give my house a bad name."

That was interesting, but understandable. No one wanted to be near a place where the unmentionable had occurred.

I raised an eyebrow. "I'd like to take another look at that room. If it's a nice one, I might know someone who's looking to change digs."

Mama Gerda grudgingly put the broom aside and led the way up the stairs.

The room didn't improve when seen in full daylight. The walls were plain plaster. The one window was clear glass, with a simple cloth over it to catch the draft. Nothing to break the starkness, not even a color print of Mata Diva or Buda-Ganesha on the wall. No reading material, either, not even a cheap adventure mag or a gossip-sheet.

I scanned the walls for anything that looked like an opening, maybe a hole covered over by plaster. There was nothing, not a crack, not a break. The floorboards looked solid, nothing to indicate a possible hiding place. I tapped the floor with my heel to make sure. No hollowness, no sign of a hidey-hole.

The table and chair were four-square, no drawers or pads. The alcohol lamp was one of the most practical. You'd never know anyone had lived in this room.

I looked at the bare pegs sticking out of the wall next to the window.

"Where are his duds? I thought I saw a tasty selection when I came in yesterday."

"The pickers took what his friends didn't last night, after the Guards left." Mama Gerda shrugged. "Emil wasn't going to need them anymore. I wasn't going to keep them myself, not even to sell at the Thieves' Market. Bad spirits cling to them."

I checked the bed. "Where's the mattress? And the straw pallet?"

"The Sanitary Squad took both of them away. Said they were full of insects, a breeding-ground for disease."

And well it might be true, but the Sanitary Squad wasn't usually so quick to clear out a dwelling in Fishmarket, no matter how filthy it got. Clearly, someone important wanted that book, enough to bribe the Dark Ones to go after it. That is, assuming it was tucked into that bedding, and I'd missed it the first time I looked for it.

I gave it some more thought, standing in the middle of the bare room while the drumming and jingling and tootling outside grew louder and more intense.

What if Jakki had found the book? If he thought it had some value, he'd want to sell it to whoever hired Emil to get it in the first place, but who was that? Did Jakki know who it was? Too many ifs.

I decided I would chase down the Sanitary Squad, then find Jakki. He had to be somewhere close, in Fishmarket or the Waterfront. I'd catch up with him once I'd dealt with the bedding.

Downstairs, the musicians had been joined by four joyboys, five females in colorful gauze skirts and headwraps, a gaggle of youngsters in various states of tatters,

77

and four hardbodies led by Brutus. All yelling in assorted Pangkoti dialects.

I didn't have to know Pangkoti to figure out what was going on. The hardbodies didn't like being woken at the break of dawn by bells and drums. The priests were determined to invoke whatever deities they worshiped on behalf of Emil the Joyboy. The rest of them were on hand to enjoy the show.

The instrumental and choral portion of the worship died down. Brutus addressed the two priests in Lorran.

"We're trying to sleep. Go away, and take your prayers somewhere else, where they will do more good. Emil was a foolish lad, and he met a sorry end."

"By you!" someone in the crowd yelled.

"Not by me!" Brutus retorted. "By someone who uses a cord. I use a knife!"

"His spirit is uneasy," a yellow-draped priest stated.

"Then let those whose business it is to find out things do their work," Brutus told him. "At least they do it quietly. They do not disturb honest folk who deserve a rest. Go to your temples, and let us alone!"

"Impious one!" The red faction had to get their coin's-worth in. "Emil was generous to Buda-Ganesha. He gave to the poor of the temples. He must be properly mourned."

"He was a faithful follower of Mata Diva!" The yellow-clad priest insisted. "He would never be so foolish as to depend on Buda-Ganesha for protection. Mata Diva gives strength to warriors!"

"Emil was no warrior," Brutus countered both of them. "Mata Diva was not his friend."

"He gave to the soup kitchen," the yellow priest insisted. "He came to worship."

"He cared for the destitute," the red priest added. "Buda-Ganesha loved him for his charity."

"*We* mourn him," one of the ragged youngsters spoke up. "He let us stay in his rooms when he wasn't there. Jakki said it was all right, that we could be there, no matter what Mama Gerda said." He folded his arms and glared at the caretaker.

One of the hardbodies behind Brutus took a turn. "Go mourn him somewhere else, and let the rest of us alone!"

"In the name of Buda-Ganesha…"

"In the name of Mata Diva…"

I worked my way around the crowd, grabbed Brutus by the arm, and dragged him into the narrow space between two houses.

"Brutus, did you get the boffin to his digs?"

He pulled his arm out of my grasp. "I sat with him on that carrier all the way around the Central Plaza to the Advanced Academy station. It took forever, and he was fussing all the way, telling me how he should have stayed with the ones who invited him, it was bad manners to run out on them. I saw him get off."

"Did he go into his lodgings?" I persisted.

"I suppose he did. There was someone waiting for him at the carrier station. Zac seemed to know the fella, so I figured he'd met one of his boffin friends. The two of them walked away together.

"The Transporteer told me he'd let me stay on the carrier so I didn't have to get off and then on and pay another fare. I didn't see why not. Did I do something wrong?"

I wasn't sure. Something felt dicey, but I couldn't say what.

"No, you did what you were told to do. Did you get a good look at the one who met him?"

"Too dark. It was a male, though. Tall, broad, and wore some kind of big hat."

I thought this over while Brutus returned to the dispute and I faded back, away from what looked like a riot in the making.

I just wished the Pangkoti would solve their religious differences in an orderly fashion, without drums, whistles, or fistfights. Religion in Lorr is usually something kept to oneself. If you find someone with like beliefs, so much the better. Otherwise, philosophy is for Academics. The Founders put it into the Regs—There is to be no one religion in Lorr.

I started along the main thoroughfare of the sector, passing the local Guardhouse on my way. It was not much more than a shack, with two Guards lounging in front, sipping their morning clet.

"There's something brewing over there," I told them, nodding in the direction of the noise. "Could be the Pangkoti are having a small religious festival. Or maybe it's a riot. I can't tell one from the other."

The larger Guard, a fairskin female of middle years and considerable heft, grimaced. It could have been the taste of the clet, or the thought of having to do some work.

"We'd better sort it out," she said, with a sigh.

Her male cohort, a bit younger and considerably thinner, agreed. They headed toward the brewing fight. If nothing else, the presence of City Guards might stop blood from being shed.

I continued along Fishmarket Way. The two Pangkoti temples, one on either side of the road, were open for business, each sponsoring a food station. Mata Diva's worshippers were mostly male—pedi-shaw drivers, from the look of them—whereas Buda-Ganesha attracted females. You'd think it would be the other way around, but there's no understanding of religion.

I passed countless Vikk-shops, cletstalls, and food shops, interspersed with small craftsmen's studios where baskets were woven and pottery jars were made and sold. So much for the conflict between the Guilds.

I made a quick stop at Drushka's Vikk-shop. I'd helped the Pangkoti refugee a while back, finding out what had happened to her spouse and getting her some concessions from the Vikk organization as compensation. Now, she was one of my main sources of information about the Pangkoti community.

Drushka's spouse had left her with a conspicuous token of his love. From the look of it, she was going to add to the population of Lorr fairly soon. She was glad to see me, but wasn't very informative about the joyboys. Or the street lizards, either.

"I do not deal with such persons," she told me, with much jingling of bracelets and chains. "They do not come to this shop."

"But you know Jakki," I pointed out. "He was hooked up with Emil."

"Jakki is very troubled. He comes to me for help, but he does not take my advice. He listens to the wrong people. He does not heed the words of the Nameless One, to endure this life in hopes of a better one." Drushka sighed. "As for Emil, he followed the path of Mata Diva, not the Nameless One. It is said his mother was Pangkoti, not his father. He used his body for personal gain. He gave bad advice to Jakki, encouraging him to lead his friends into evil."

"Let me know if Jakki shows up."

"What has happened to him?" Druska was visibly worried.

"He's got in over his head. He may have seen or heard something that makes him a target. You heard what happened to Emil."

Drusha shuddered, and made the Desert Folk's sign to avert evil.

"If Jakki comes to you, send him on to me," I told her. I considered buying more clet-powder, but decided against it. I didn't know how long I'd be chasing the Sanitary Squad, and I didn't want to be burdened with a jar.

I continued my stroll through Fishmarket. All the while, I kept an eye out for the Sanitary Squad, supposedly making their rounds with the Dark Ones' pedicart. I saw empty bins outside the shops, a sign they'd been past; but every time I thought I spotted them, they turned another corner.

I caught a glimpse of blue-clad figures heaving bins and baskets into the back of a pedi-cart. I kept an eye peeled for Jakki, but I didn't see him, or anyone like him, not even one of those street lizards. I decided they must all be watching the show at the joyboys' lodging, and slogged on.

Ahead of me loomed the old brick buildings once used for manufactures, now taken over by the Dark Ones. And behind them…the discard pits, where just maybe I'd find what I was looking for.

I could stay in Fishmarket, comb through the alleys, and try to find Jakki. Or I could forge ahead, confront the office drones guarding the Dark Ones' Temple of Healing, and find the pallet. I decided Jakki could keep for now. He'd turn up, one way or another.

If he'd found the book, he'd want to get a buyer. If he hadn't, no point looking for him. He'd vanish into the side streets and alleys, just another of the youngsters scrabbling to survive in the general population of Lorr.

I crossed the short bridge over the stream where Fishmarket Way turned into Industrial Way. A line of twisted trees marked the border between the districts, but I could tell by the change in housing I had crossed a less visible barrier. There was a world of difference between Fishmarket people and Industrial people, and it wasn't just the houses and the food. It was the attitude, the smug righteousness of Industrial, that made me want to stick someone in the eye.

I had taken coin to find the book. The best lead I had was that scroungy bedding, and that was headed for the recycle pits in Industrial. Like it or not, that was where I had to go.

ii

I do not like the Industrial Sector. It's not just the looming buildings, the Temple of Healing, and the Advanced Academy, one at either end of Industrial Way. They'd housed the factories that made Lorr the manufacturing center for New Earth until their poisonous by-products led to a major uprising by the mechs who had to endure them.

That, in turn, led to the reversal of policy by Admin. The factories had been moved safely away from the city center, across the river to Flatlands or southward to the Pangkot border three generations ago. After strenuous efforts, their waste products had been eliminated from the environment so that Lorrans once again had clean water to drink and fresh air to breathe.

The housing here isn't as threatening as the tangled alleys and weird corners of Fishmarket, or as intimidating as the blank walls that hide the mansions on Striver's Hill and Arriver's Hill. You could even say the residences are good-looking, in their way.

The Second Ship manufacturers built them in straight rows, one connected to the other, for both the mechanicals who did the heavy work and the technicians who directed them. They equipped them with all the proper amenities, such as wiring for electrics, water pipes in every house, and sewer connections to dispense waste. Nothing like the squalor just over the stream in Fishmarket. Boring, neat and regulated, like the machines the former occupants tended.

But when the factories went over the river, so did the people who ran them. Now, the houses are hot properties, taken over by the Dark Ones connected with the Temple of Healing and the boffins of the Advanced Academy for their personnel.

It's those people that get up my nose. All of them have this smug air about them, that they know something lesser mortals don't. Whether they're med-techs, cleaners, even students at the Advanced Academy, they act as if they are superior simply because they can face the unthinkable and not flinch. Death has no effect on Industrial people. They live with it all the time.

But Eyeing means going places I don't like, including the Dark One's Temple, a huge brick-and-stone structure with tall windows that dominates the rest of the district. A space in front of the Temple has been cleared for hand-carts, pedi-carts, pedi-shaws, and official skimmers, with racks for the two-wheels ridden by the office drones and med-techs toiling inside busily keeping Lorr healthy and safe.

It's a heavy burden on the Dark Ones, to hear them tell it, and they do tell it, loudly, through the posts. There are always disputes in the City Council, claims from this or that Guild that the Dark Ones are interfering with business.

On their part, the Dark Ones claim they are responsible to their deity, Saint Hygeia, for keeping Lorr clean and free of disease and pollutants.

The Grocer's Guild yells about Dark Ones constantly monitoring food supplies. The Construction Guild isn't happy when Dark Ones send inspectors to make a fuss about unsafe conditions in living quarters. Transporteers grumble about Dark Ones regulating fuels, claiming they can't always rely on wind to get their ships to and from northern and southern ports on schedule.

No one wants to think about what happens to the deceased, once the Dark Ones carry them off to the other side of Lorr, far away from the rest of the city, to be reduced to their component chemicals.

But the Dark Ones staff the Shrines to Hygeia, two or three per district, with med-techs in attendance to treat injuries, medicate minor illnesses, and provide care for infants' and children's ailments. I've been grateful for their services from time to time.

The Temple of Healing deals with the more serious life-and-death struggles and severe injuries. So, I shouldn't complain about all those clerks and office drones who support the ones in the Shrines. Someone has to keep the records and enter them into the Big Black Box.

As for the ones who actually cut into living flesh… the less aid about them, the better.

While I stood weighing my options, I spotted the San-itary Squad pedi-cart just ahead. I'd finally caught up with it.

I loped after it, shouting, "Oyo! Stop!"

The driver either didn't hear me or didn't want to understand. He headed for the near end of the Temple of Healing, and a gap in the shrubbery surrounding it.

A waist-high fence blocked casual passers-by from entering. A sign in Lorran and Pangkoti lettering read:

KEEP OUT

ENTRANCE FORBIDDEN BY ORDER OF ADMINISTRATION OF NEW EARTH

The pedi-cart driver blew his klaxon. A blue-clad mech opened a gate in the fence and the pedi-cart drove in. I sprinted after and slid through just as the mech closed the gate.

"Official business for the Guild," I panted, and ran after the pedi-cart. I didn't say which Guild, just hoped the guard would assume Fatsos and ask no more questions.

Having never been here before, I stopped short as I realized the Temple surmounted a steep cliff with a sheer drop to the beach below. A flight of stairs had been cut into the limestone cliff, a rope anchored to posts set into the open edge, the minimal safety measure. I scanned the space below the stairs. Was it worth my while to go down, or should I stay where I was and take my chances with the drones in the Temple.

The beach stretched towards the estuary— the tide was out, leaving bunches of seaweed here and there between the pools where small creatures lived in and around the rocks. A few people squatted around the pools. I had no idea why, or what they were doing. My attention was drawn to the apparatus creaking alongside the stairs.

A squad of Dark mechs was loading the Sanitary Squad pedi-cart onto a platform. A system of ropes and pulleys, powered by a small engine that emitted gusts of evil-smelling smoke, lowered it to the beach.

I peered over the cliff to see what would happen to the contents of that pedi-cart. A line of them stretched along the beach in front of a set of huge metal bins. Each bin bore a label and a symbol for its contents: Metal, Glass, Fabric, Paper.

More blue-clad Dark mechs swarmed over each pedi-cart, removing anything inorganic and placing it into the appropriate bin. Organic matter was tossed onto the beach, to be devoured by the pteros or crustaceans in the sand.

Beyond the breakers I could see the barges, ready to come in at high tide to carry the larger bits away to the factories to be reduced to their component elements and recycled into more goods to be sold somewhere. All part of the Economy of New Earth.

I stood at the top of the cliff. No point in trying to get anyone's attention on the beach—their eyes were on their work, and they probably couldn't see me, anyway. My ears were battered by the squawking pteros, the engine's clank and roar, and the wind whistling against the cliff face. The stink of rotting vegetation and salt water assaulted my nasal passages.

I looked around for another means of descent. Surely, all these people didn't climb up and down this staircase to get to their work? The loading platform was already on its way up, but I didn't have the time to argue with the mechs who ran it to get me down to the beach. If I wanted to find that book before it was tossed away, I'd have to go down those stairs.

I am not good at heights. I don't even like skimmers, although they're the fastest way to get from one place to another.

I tried to convince myself I didn't have to do this. I didn't even know if the bedding was there, or if the book was in the bedding. Then, I caught a glimpse of a tangle of cloth and straw being heaved out of one pedi-cart.

I edged onto the stairs, holding the rope with one hand, taking one step at a time, carefully placing my feet on the slippery steps. I was halfway down when I thought I heard a footstep somewhere above me.

I couldn't be sure. Between the clanking of the machinery and the squawking pteros, my ears weren't able to focus, and I couldn't tell who it was by scent, either.

Before I could turn, I felt a strong hand shove the middle of my back. I stumbled and started to fall, holding onto the rope railing with one hand, trying to fend off the attacker with the other. I swung outward, nearly smashing against the cliff wall as I waved my free hand wildly to steady myself. I made contact with the cliff face, still clinging to the rope. I swung back to the steps, scrambling for a foothold.

Someone kicked my feet away. I grabbed at the rope with the other hand. Now I could maneuver with both hands on the rope, kicking out again to find the stairs. I tried to see who it was who'd attacked me, but all I got was a glimpse of a blue-clad back hustling down the stairs and onto the beach.

I thought I heard footsteps, something smacking against the stone, as I managed to get a toehold in a crack in the stone. Finally stabilized, I swung forward and heaved myself back onto the stairs.

Someone else was on those stairs behind me. I tensed, waiting for another attack. It didn't come. Instead, someone grabbed me by the shoulders, steadied me on the stairs, and helped me down to the beach.

I was still shaking when I felt sand under my feet instead of slippery rock. Someone prized my hands off the rope and handed me a cloth.

"Use this."

I wiped smuts out of my eyes, blew my nose, and muttered some kind of thanks.

"Think nothing of it. Us Eyes have to stick together."

I looked into the face of my savior—Reg Bonwit.

iii

"What are you doing here?" I asked. Not the most gracious response to someone who may have just saved my life…if he wasn't the one who'd pushed me in the first place.

"Following orders," Reg said. "Eye Hunt wanted information relating to the case we're on, and I was on my way to the Advanced Academy to get it when I saw you heading for the stairs. Didn't you see the loading platform?"

"Sure I did. It was going up, I wanted to go down. And there's all this smoke." I managed a grin, and jerked my head upward towards the ancient engine wheezing away amid the ropes and pulleys.

Reg applied another nose wipe to his own face. "I thought those old fuel-burners were discarded when the factories got moved out of Lorr."

"This one wasn't." I blew soot out of my nose, and regretted it. There was more than just smoke in the air. "You didn't happen to see anyone leaving when you came down those stairs?"

"Not anyone going up."

"Then he must have gone down," I concluded.

"He?" Reg asked. "How can you be sure?"

"The size and shape of the hand on my back," I stated firmly. "And I don't know any large *females* who'd want to shove me off a cliff. At least, not right now," I amended.

"Not even this one?"

By this time we had reached the bottom of the staircase. Reg nodded toward the mechs' leader, a loud-voiced female who looked at the sun and announced, "Midday break!"

Work stopped as a large handcart was lowered on the platform. The mechs clustered around it, ready for whatever edibles were being distributed.

By this time the med-tech in charge, a hefty middle-aged male in regulation Dark Ones blue spotted Reg and me.

"Oyo! What are you doing here? This is a restricted zone!"

I fished out one of my outdated Admin sigils and hoped he wouldn't examine it too closely.

"I have permission to examine these bins for an item that may have been discarded accidentally."

"And you?" The tech glared at Reg

"Another errand, but I'm with Eye Drach."

"What sort of item?" The tech frowned at the two of us.

"A book," I said. "About the size of two hands. Bound in leather."

"What makes you think it's here?" The supervisor wasn't charmed by either my bland smile or Reg's smirk.

"It was last in the hands of a certain person who may have hidden it in some bedding that was just picked up by the Sanitary Squad," I told him. "I saw the straw pallet going past in the pedi-cart just before I…missed my footing on the stairs." I decided not to accuse anyone of trying to murder me. Not yet.

"You didn't see anyone else coming down?" Reg asked, scanning the busy scene.

"I got better things to do than watch the stairs," the tech grumbled. "And anything like a book would get taken out of the cart before it even gets here. Our people don't just throw things out. We sift the large items before we bring them to recycling. You want it, you go through the Central Office." He pointed to the platform. "You can take the lift."

I considered questioning the mechs directly, then decided it would be a waste of their time and mine. They were all intent on getting their lunch. A giant reptile could have come up from the sea, and they wouldn't notice. The people clustered around the tide pools were too far from the stairs to have seen anything, so no point asking them, either.

I shrugged and headed for the lift platform. A patch of greenery at the base of the cliff caught my eye—writhing tendrils, tiny white florets, and long red pods.

"Vampire vines?" I turned to the tech. "Did you know they were there? They're supposed to be removed if they take root."

"They keep the rodents and felines down," the tech replied. "We burn them for fuel. The beans aren't bad for eating."

"Considering what's in them?" I shuddered. Vampire vines are one of the native predators on New Earth, along with sundews and sticker trees. This particular patch had an unusual shape. I looked again, with growing horror as I realized what it was.

"Dark Tech," I said slowly, "I think there is something under that vampire vine that is not a feline or a rodent."

Reg added, "Don't touch it with bare hands. Get something sharp to pull it out."

The tech in charge hesitated—the vine was writhing in full feeding mode. Then, he gulped and yelled orders. The mechs stopped eating. There was a lot of discussion, in various dialects of Lorran Standard. Finally, a large female mech grabbed a pole from the nearest pedicart and started scything the vines away from whatever they were feeding on.

The first swipe revealed a male torso, blood oozing from where the vine's suckers had penetrated the skin.

The second swipe got the vine away from its neck. The third revealed the face, what there was of it, after the vine's suckers had attacked the soft tissues of the eyes and lips..

"Merciful Founders, that's Zac!" I blurted.

And that's where I disgraced myself by losing what little I'd had to eat before I set out.

iv

Reg sat me down on the bottom step while the tech supervisor sent for reinforcements. There was a ferocious argument between him and the mech female as to what to do with the late Zac Garber. The tech insisted protocol called for keeping him where he was. The mech pointed out that, if they did, the vampire vines would continue to leach his vital fluids, making it difficult for the Medical Examiners to find out exactly what had caused his demise.

Neither tech nor mechs wanted to get anywhere near that vampire vine without a hazmat suit. They argued that with the supervisor until he agreed to their demands.

Finally, the Tech Supervisor sent one of the mechs upward on the platform to notify the Dark Masters that a body had been found. The others chopped away enough vines so they could yank said body out of the voracious greenery onto the sand.

That gave me enough time to control my involuntary nervous system. I was still shuddering when they got Zac out of the vines. I took one more look, and noticed a red line across his throat.

Then, a skimmer landed on the beach in a spray of sand and salt water. Out came Captain Sara Atterson, along with two Guards and Dark One Kelvin. The platform descended, carrying a squad of white-clad miscellaneous Dark Ones and one tall old male in the blue robes of a Dark Master.

The Dark Ones gathered around Zac's remains, arguing loudly. One of the mechs had run after them with a container of water so they could wash their hands before touching the victim.

Atterson spotted Reg and me sitting on the bottom stair.

"Oyo, Eye Drach. I should have guessed you'd be here." She looked across the beach. The tide was coming in, gradually narrowing the expanse of sand. "What can you tell me that I don't already know?"

"The male in the vines is a Contramonter boffin, name of Zac Garber," I informed her. "A student at the Advanced Academy."

"I said, what I don't know," Atterson said. "I've already been told who he was. What I want to know is, what are you doing here, and what else do you know about Boffin Garber?"

"He was the client who wanted me to find a book for him," I said. "I was following a lead yesterday, when I saw you at Fishmarket. It looks like I was right—the joyboy had it, but with him gone…who knows?"

Atterson considered that, then addressed Reg. "And what about you, Eye Bonwit? What brings you to the recycling beach?"

"I was on my way to interview someone at the Advanced Academy regarding a client of Independent Eye Hunt when I saw Eye Drach was in trouble. I went to her assistance, as a friend would. Independent Eyes have to stick together." Reg was back to his usual smarmy self. I didn't believe him for a minute. For all I knew, he was the one who'd pushed me.

"This book." Atterson dismissed Reg and turned back to me. "Is it valuable?"

"Not very, except to Friend Zac, and whoever wanted to get it away from him.

Atterson's eyes narrowed. "And what's so interesting about this book?"

"No idea, but someone wanted it enough to pay Emil to seduce our friend there, then sent a hardbody to get it from Emil," I said. "Whatever's in it is worth a lot to someone, but don't ask me who or why, because I don't know."

Atterson turned back to Reg. "And your errand at the Advanced Academy? What has that got to do with this book? Atterson turned to Reg.

"Nothing, so far as I know. Unless what's in the book has to do with coal mining."

"It might," I suggested. "That's what Boffin Zac told me he was going to lecture about."

Atterson frowned. "Is that enough to kill for?"

Reg shrugged. "Like Eye Drach, I have no ideas on the subject. I was supposed to fetch one of the boffins from the Advanced Academy to Eye Hunt's house, to instruct her on the ins and outs of coal production. To find out more, ask Eye Hunt, not me."

Atterson muttered something under her breath, not complimentary, about Independent Eye Julian Hunt. "Drach, when did you see this youngster last?"

I couldn't very well say I hadn't seen him, not with Reg there to contradict me.

"Last night. He was at Smokey Joe's with Gorgeous Gyorgi Delrey and some of his pals. They caused a bit of a ruckus. I got young Zac out of there before the Guards came to quiet things down. You've probably got the report on your desk right now."

Atterson grimaced. "I don't get those reports anymore. I'm on Special Squad, remember? No one tells me anything. What about you, Bonwit? What do you know about this boffin?"

"Less than Pola," Reg said. "Eye Hunt is looking into something for the Contramont Miners' Trade Delegation. They're sponsoring Boffin Zac Garber at the Advanced Academy. One of their younger members saw him chatting up Gyorgi Delrey. He was afraid the youngster might be giving away some information that could be used against them in the current negotiations with the Delrey Banking interests, told his senior, and the senior told Hunt. Eye Hunt had me following the lad, keeping an eye on him, to see just how much of this was gossip and how much it had to do with some missing funds we're tracking down."

That explained why Reg had been consorting with us lowlifes at Smokey Joe's.

"And what happened to Garber last night?"

Atterson wouldn't let it go. I took up the tale.

"After I got him out of Smokey Joe's. I put Zac on the carrier, with one of the Flatlands Force to guard him. I told him to get back to the hostel where he was staying." It suddenly hit me. "Merciful Founders, I led that lad to his death!"

"What are you saying?" she asked sharply.

"The Fatso, Brutus, the one who lives near the joy-boys' lodgings, was with him on the carrier, but left him at the station. Or so he told me this morning."

"When was that?" Atterson produced a small note-book and stylus to make notes.

"When he left Smokey Joe's, or when I saw him this morning?" I hedged.

"Last night." she gritted out, visibly holding her temper in check.

"I don't carry a timepiece," I said. "But it was well after sunset when Zac and Brutus got on the carrier. Can't say how far the night had gone, but it was moon-dark."

Reg fished a standard twelve-hour pocket model timepiece out of his trou pocket.

"I'd place the time between seventh and eighth hour. I saw the boffin and the guard mount the carrier together."

"This Brutus...Isn't he the Pangkoti who was cited for nonconsensual intimacy? The one who was on Ishka Kunine's ship?" Atterson frowned.

"Brutus is what he goes by in Lorr," I admitted. "And he's changed his employers. He's now with the Flat-lands Force, and he's a member of the Assassins' Guild, in good standing."

"That means nothing. We keep a sharp eye on all of Kunine's castaways," Atterson said. "For all we know, they're still loyal to Pangkot. If he's a big hardbody with tats on his arms, I saw him hanging around the joyboys' digs yesterday. Someone in the crowd pointed him out as the perpetrator of the deed."

"That's Brutus, all right, but he swears by the goddess of Pangkot he didn't do it, and I believe him. It's not his style."

"That's not for you to decide, Drach. I think I'll have a little chat with Flatlands Force Brutus. Even if he's not longing for Pangkot, he just might still be working for the Delreys, with or without Guild sanction. Thank you for your information, Eye Drach, Eye Bonwit. Now let the City Guards hand this. It's what the Administration pays us to do. Keep out of it."

She turned back to the gang gathered around the late Zac Garber and started in on the mechs. A few of the crabbers joined the group to see what was going on.

I drew Reg out of the way of the crowd.

"She's wrong. Brutus didn't do this, any more than he did Emil. He's a knife man, doesn't use a cord."

Reg had other troubles on his mind. "I'm not looking forward to telling Eye Hunt about this. The Contramont Miners thought the world of Friend Zac. He was a shining star, according to Elder Mackintosh.

"They don't sponsor many students for the Lorr Advanced Academy, mostly sending their bright young lads to Port Chicago. This lad, Zac, must have been considered something really special to get a scholarship and passage all the ways to Lorr."

"Fee M'Farr won't be pleased when he hears of it, either," I added. "He hates it when some amateur takes a life instead of hiring an assassin who'll do it properly." I looked up at the stairs and shuddered at the thought of climbing them. "Is there any other way back up?"

One of the mechs saw my distress. "You can take the lift," he offered.

Reg and I slogged over the sand to the platform. He helped me onto the thing, and we hung on to the ropes while someone on the cliff above winched us aloft. It wasn't much better than the stairs, swaying back and forth, but at least something else was fighting the pull of New Earth's gravity instead of just my legs.

We reached the top of the cliff and passed through the gate to the plaza in front of the Temple.

"What next?" Reg looked around for a pedi-shaw. "I've got to report to Eye Hunt. If you're heading back to Entertainment Row, I can take you as far as Arriver's Hill."

"I'll take the carrier," I demurred. "I have to alert Master Assassin M'Farr that one of his new recruits is about to be picked up for overstepping his authority. And I'm not going back to my digs just yet. I've got to look in at my office, see if anything new has come up."

Before we reached Industrial Way, a trio of males in Contramont garb confronted us.

"You! You're the one works for Independent Eye Julian Hunt?"

Reg admitted it was he. "Independent Eye Reg Bonwit. How may I be of assistance?" He sounded like a shop clerk in one of the pricey boutiques on the Grand Boulevard.

"You can tell us what happened to our dear friend and colleague Zacharias!"

That was the largest male—stout, brown beard down to the top of the bib, head topped with the Contramonter broad-brimmed straw hat.

The smallest of the lot, a wrinkled character with a sparse white beard piped up. "We were summoned here from our residence by a messenger from the Dark Ones. He said young Zac has met with an accident of some kind."

"As far as we know, he went over the cliff, into a patch of vampire vines," I said. "The Dark Ones are working on him now, to see if it was purposeful or accidental."

"Purposeful?"

"Do you mean…murder?" The third Contramonter, long and stringy, somewhere in age between the other two, was aghast.

"I don't think Boffin Zac was planning to walk off the cliff," I said.

"And there's a railing just to make sure no one trips and falls over." Reg pointed to the gap between two of the Academy buildings. 'I'm inclined to agree with Eye Drach. Someone must have helped Friend Zac over that cliff."

"This is terrible!" Brown Beard blustered. The other two made noises of agreement as they moved away.

"Friends," I said. "If I may have your attention?"

They stopped and turned to glare at me, no doubt astonished that a mere female should dare to speak in their august presence without permission.

"I am Independent Eye Pola Drach. Boffin Zacharias Garber came to my office yesterday and asked me to find something for him. I took his coin, but I never finished the job. This puts me in a difficult position since, as the Regulations of Lorr clearly state, there are severe penalties for not fulfilling the terms of a contract."

Brown Beard frowned down at me. "What is this about a contract? Zacharias did not tell me of any contract when we last spoke."

"When was that?" Reg asked.

"Yesterday, in the hour before sundown. I met him at the Strangers Hostel."

"Was that when you told him to go slumming with Gorgeous Gyorgi Delrey?" Now we were getting somewhere! "Are you the one he called Elder Mackintosh?"

"I am Hosea Mackintosh, Elder of Contramont." He looked me over.

I wasn't at my best, after the scramble on the cliff stairs, but I didn't deserve that sneer of contempt. I put it down to Contramont prejudice. Typical Second Ship stuff.

The First-Ship Founders didn't make a fuss about gender roles—if a job needed doing, it got done by whoever could do it best. Second Ship had a lot more restrictions, and it got worse when they started spreading out and establishing new settlements with their own ways of doing things. Contramont is one of the more extreme gender-separate settlements, but Norlander females are just as nasty to males as Contramonter males are to females.

"Elder Mackintosh, what am I to do about this contract?" I persisted. "I've taken coin, but I haven't finished the job. Do I still owe it to Boffin Zacharias to find the item he asked me to find?"

Elder Mackintosh looked to the other two, then back at me.

"Your contract is nullified with the demise of our dear friend Zacharias," he told me. "You need not worry about penalties. Go about your other business, and do not bother us again. The journal you were sent to find is irrelevant."

He turned his back on me and headed toward the Temple.

"I've got to report this to The Brain," Reg said. "The pedi-shaw offer's still open. It's a long ways back to Clothier's Alley."

"I'll take the carrier," I said. "I have a few stops to make before I hit my office. As I said, Fee M'Farr will want to know about Brutus, and I want to check that contract before I close the case."

"Elder Mackintosh closed it for you," Reg said as he mounted the nearest pedi-shaw and rode off.

That's what he thinks!

I felt responsible for Zac's demise. Maybe, if I'd gone after that book last night instead of going home… if I'd gone after Jakki instead of the pallet…

But that was useless second-guessing. What had happened was done. What was *going* to happen…that was something else.

ν

So, there I was, no client in sight, dismissed by the client's superiors. I took the next carrier as far as the grim building that housed the Honorable Guild of Forgers, Assassins, Thieves, and Swindlers. Spies had probably informed Master Assassin Fee M'Farr of the unfortunate fate of Joyboy Emil; but we'd just found Boffin Zac, and his sources among the Dark Ones might not have reported to him yet.

I left word with Ratty, Fee's personal gatekeeper and trusted minion, and went on my way. It would be up to Fee M'Farr to decide if the killing of an outsider warranted his attention. Let him fight it out with Captain Atterson; I was officially off the case.

Unofficially, I still had a lot of questions I wanted answered before I closed the files.

I made it back to my office in Clothier's Alley. Jake was waiting for me.

"There's a message from Basher Bob Basheer. He wants you to contact him at Smokey Joe's as soon as possible. And you have a client," he told me. "I let him in. He looks harmless, young and skinny. He's wearing one of those new kilt things, a cheap knockoff of Guernreich's latest fad. Trying to imitate the Admin lads, no doubt."

Trust Jake to judge a person by his dress.

"If it's the street lizard I'm thinking about, he's probably gone through all my files and made off with the cashbox."

I went in and found Jakki sitting on the uncomfortable wooden chair. He jumped up as soon as he saw me.

"Eye Pola Drach! Where have you been? I have waited for you all day. I have something you want. Something you are looking for."

"You should have waited at your digs," I scolded him. "*I've* been looking for *you*. I left word with Drushka at her Vikk-shop."

"I know. When the Dark Ones came to clean Emil's room, they took my bedding away. I could not stay in that house—there are spirits there. Emil does not rest."

"I thought the priests had dealt with that."

"Emil does not care," Jakki sniveled. "He was not of Pangkot, not really. He gave coin to the priests because he liked to show how generous he was, but he did not believe in Buda-Ganesha or Mata Diva. He told me the Nameless One watches over all Humanity, the others are illusions."

I thought that over while Jakki went on.

"They did not find this thing, because I had already taken it away before they got there. Emil showed it to me and hid it in his bed, but then he was killed. I was afraid, so I took it away and put it in a safer place. Then, I went back to the house.

"The Guards were there, but they did not know about this. And you asked about it, but I did not know if I could trust you.

"So I asked Vikk-shop Drushka, and she said you helped her, that you were a good person, and I should go to you. So, I have done so."

He laid a small leatherbound book on my desk.

Founder's Faith! I'd run off my feet, nearly been thrown down stairs, and braved a patch of vampire vines for this thing, and it had been in my own office the whole time.

I picked it up, almost afraid to touch it, and riffled the pages to see what the fuss was about. It was filled with incomprehensible cramped writing in an alphabet I didn't recognize. Not Lorran, for sure, or any of the variants. Not Pangkoti, either. There were strings of standard numbers, but they meant nothing to me. There were drawings of weird apparatuses, equally meaningless.

And for this mishmash two persons were killed? It made no sense to me.

I would have to find someone else to decipher this journal. Someone who had the kind of brain that relished this sort of puzzle. Someone who would be in my debt if I handed this over to them.

I looked back at Jakki, who squirmed in the uncomfortable chair.

"Why did you bring this to me? You know there are people looking for it. The Guards, for one, and Brutus, for another. And whoever hired Emil to get it is probably willing to pay for it."

"The Guards won't pay for it. Brutus won't, either. And I don't want to give it to the one who killed Emil to get it. He might kill me, too, instead of paying for it."

106

"Good reasoning."

"Merchant Drushka from the Vikk-shop told me where your office was. She said you helped her, and you will help me if I pay you to do it."

I looked at him again. "What do you want me to do with this?" I tapped the book.

"I want to find out who killed Emil. I will trade this book for your service. You take the book, do with it what you think best, sell it to whoever will take it. Then, you find out who killed Emil."

"He meant that much to you?"

"He was my friend, but more than that, he was willing to help my other friends. He let us stay in his rooms, gave us money for food, protected us from the Guards. The Nameless One tells me I must get his killer. Find out who did this evil thing. Tell me, and I will do the rest,"

Just like a Pangkoti. Private vengeance, carried out privately. More troubles for Fee M'Farr, but not my concern.

"Very well, you're now my client. Do *not* lie to me —it will only muddle things. Start from the beginning. When did you last see Emil?"

Jakki frowned in thought. "I think it was some time after midday on the day he was killed. He came back from a meeting with his best patron, the one who was most generous. He had me set out his best outfit—the new jacket and kilt, very modern, very trendy.

"He said there was to be a very special party at one of the fine pleasure houses on Red Lantern Alley, and he had been hired to be there, to take care of someone the patron wanted to impress. He hinted there might be extra coin if he pleased the patron. He said if he did well, we would be able to move to the Artist's Sector, away from Fishmarket, with the higher-up Entertainers."

"He would take you with him?"

"I looked after him well," Jakki explained. "I ran his errands. I made sure no one disturbed him when he slept. I fetched the water from the outside faucet, kept the room clean, made sure there were no remains when my friends stayed there."

"He didn't bring, um, patrons there?" I hinted.

"Never!" Jakki stated firmly. "It was his home. He did his business elsewhere. I do not know where."

"You should register with the Servant's Guild," I suggested. "Go on. When did Emil leave for this fancy party?"

"After our evening meal," Jakki went on. "And I did not see him again until very late. I stayed up for him. Sometimes, after an evening party, he would not be himself."

"Weed or jack?" I asked. A lot of the Licensees dulled their senses with one or the other, sometimes both. Not a good combination.

Jakki squirmed again. "He smelled of weed sometimes. But not this time. He was not muzzy. He was very alert. He told me he had something that would bring us much coin, but he would not tell me what it was, only that I must say nothing about it to anyone.

"He sent me downstairs to get water to wash with. I saw him hide a book in his bedding. I went down, I got the water, I started to go back up the stairs."

He stopped for breath.

"Take your time. Think, Jakki. What did you see on the stairs?"

He closed his eyes, then opened them. "It was dark, just the light from the lantern at the door. I didn't hear anything from the people in the house—they were in their own rooms, I suppose they were asleep. There was no one on the street at the water-faucet. There may have been someone when I went down, but there were many shadows. When I had the water, I went back into the house, and then I saw the djinn."

"Was this djinn going down or coming up?"

"He was going down. He brushed past me and ran out the door."

"Did you see his face? Was it Brutus?"

Jakki shook his head. "Not so big as Brutus, not so broad in the shoulder. I could not make out his face— it was covered. I was too frightened to make a noise."

"And then what?"

"I went into our room. I saw Emil on the floor and ran out, because it is a very bad thing, to be with the dead. I went to Drushka's Vikk-shop, where she used to let me sleep before I met Emil. By then, it was nearly daylight. Drushka said to go back to tell Mama Gerda what had happened, she would send for the Guards.

"When I went back, I saw Emil was still there. That was when I took the book. I hid it in a secret place. I went back to see what was happening until I heard the Guards coming. The rest you know."

That put Emil's time of demise somewhere just short of daybreak. If Brutus was to be believed, he didn't go into the house until well after dawn.

I turned the book over in my hands.

"Do you have a place to stay? Somewhere private, not the joyboys' lodging?"

"Merchant Drushka said I could help her in her shop," Jakki said. "She will let me stay with her."

"Go there, stay out of sight," I ordered. "Leave the book with me—I'll get it to someone who knows how to read it."

"Not the Guards! They will not help. They do not care for male Licensees."

"No, not the Guards. Someone very clever," I assured him.

He made the Pangkoti blessing sign and slid out the door, just another street lizard in the teeming crowd, mingling with the shoppers on the Grand Boulevard.

I looked through the book once again. I could see someone with tech knowledge might get some use out of the drawings of complicated machinery, but the rest was a mystery. I knew who'd enjoy solving it, though... a regular Brain

vi

So, I was back on the job, with a different client and a new question to answer: Who killed Joyboy Emil, and why?

It had been a long day, with another long night ahead of me. I needed sustenance and a bit of pampering before setting out on another night's Eyeing. Food I'd get at Fletcher's, and pampering at the baths.

But before that I had one more chore to do.

I tucked the book under my jacket and headed out, through Clothier's Alley into the afternoon ruck of the Grand Boulevard. I double-checked the Posts at the intersection. Nothing new on the status of the Contramont Miners, nothing at all about either Zac or Emil. Mysterious deaths were something Admin did not want the good citizens of Lorr to know about, not until they could present a finished case, with the culprit caught and on the way to punishment.

The book under my jacket seemed to weigh me down. I tried to sense whether I was being followed, but Ficus's gift had worn off. The sounds battering my ears were the usual ones of midafternoon—chatter of humans going about their daily business, creak and rattle of pedishaws and two-wheels, clang of the carrier bell. Nothing unusual, nothing to get my guard up.

I did notice several young males in kilts and ragged jackets lurking on street corners, ready to snatch a package from an unwary shopper; but that was to be expected. Sanctioned Thieves were an occupational hazard for shoppers on the Grand Boulevard. The unwary might lose their purchases, but they could always retrieve them at the Thieves' Market.

I stopped at Arriver's Hill and looked upwards towards the row of houses, originally built for the Administrators of the First Ship now ensconced in their mountain lairs. Arriver's Hill had been taken over by the middle tier—the advocates and magistrates who actually ran the city. They let the merchants and bankers flaunt their wealth on Striver's Hill, trying to outdo each other with gaudy furnishings and outrageously expensive artwork. The folks on Arriver's Hill knew their power, and didn't need to splash it around.

I knocked at the door two houses up the row. A panel slid back, an eye peeked out. The door opened to reveal Reg Bonwit, freshly groomed and ready for another night of Eyeing.

"Pola?" He let me into the vestibule.

"Reg. I have something the Brain might be interested in."

"Eye Hunt is up in the plant room," he told me.

I knew she spent two hours in the morning, two in the afternoon for botanical research.

"It's you I came to see."

"Come on in, then." He showed me to a small room next to the vestibule, not the large library where Hunt did business. "Haven't you had enough punishment for one day?"

"And all for this." I fished the book from under my jacket.

He whistled in astonishment. "Where did that come from?"

"From someone who got it from Joyboy Emil," I told him. "It's my fee for finding Emil's killer."

Reg's eyebrow went up. "Really? I thought that was settled. It was a Sanctioned Assassin's kill, nothing for anyone to look into. Atterson's convinced it was the hard-body from Smokey Joe's…What was his name?

112

"Brutus," I said. "But he couldn't have done it. I've got a witness who says he saw the body before sun-up. Timing's wrong." I handed the book to Reg. "I've had a look through this, but I can't make out the writing. It looks like some kind of code. I'm betting Eye Hunt can figure it out."

"So you bring it here, to the Brain, out of the kindness of your heart?"

"You probably saved my life today. This pays the debt. Besides, it's safer here than in my office, and I don't want it in my digs."

"Especially if it's so hot it burns anyone who touches it," Reg added with a grin. "Allright, I'll give it to the Brain when she gets down from her plant session. It'll be something new for her to play with."

I left with a lighter heart. What with all those advocates and magistrates in residence, Arriver's Hill was well-guarded. Whatever secrets that journal held would be kept safe until The Brain decided to reveal them.

Now all I had to do was find out who'd had it in for Joyboy Emil, and keep Brutus out of the clutches of the City Guard.

I mooched down Arriver's Hill, hopped on the next carrier, and rode cheerfully back to my digs. I had time for a quick snack at Fletcher's and a visit with Ficus before I went to the baths. I needed refreshing, and I wanted a word with someone who could give me more information on joyboys than I already had.

CHASING EMIL

MIDAFTERNOON IS A SLOW TIME AT THE BATHS. THE new constructions in Flatlands are equipped with full plumbing, so the office drones and shop clerks can do their daily ablutions at home instead of dipping and soaking with the general population. The artists tend to do their bathing in the early morning or late afternoon. Licensees come and go, but today, they mostly went. So, I pretty much had the place to myself.

I dropped my clothes at the cleaners' station to be refreshed, then went to the showers and pool. I scrubbed the smoke and grime off, took a quick rinse, and draped myself in one of the robes provided. Then I stepped over to the grooming section, where hair and nails are clipped and shaped.

There, I found Angie lounging at his stand, tall and sleek, dark skin, tight-cropped hair thinning at the top. He's one of the best hairdressers on Entertainment Row, sought after by actors, singers, and top-notch licensees. He knows everyone and everything that goes on in front of the stage as well as behind the scenes. If he didn't know about Emil, he'd know someone who did.

"Pola Drach!" He greeted me in a tone of distress. "What have you been doing to yourself? I wish you'd let me tint that mess on your head."

"I like my hair the way it is," I said. "It works with my skin tone."

"It's very beige," Angie scolded me. "I could brighten it to a true blond, one that would get you noticed."

"I don't want to be noticed," I reminded him. "I don't need a clip right now. I need some information."

Angie looked around, saw no one was watching us, and leaned closer.

"Is this about that dreadful thing that happened in Fishmarket?"

"I've been asked to look into it," I admitted. "This Emil…a joyboy, I hear."

"Licensed sex worker," Angie corrected me.

"Ever work with him?"

"Professionally or personally?" Angie smirked.

"His or yours?" I countered.

Angie looked hurt. "I do not pay for intimacy. I don't have to. As for Emil, he did not come to my stand for hairdressing. He preferred the male side of the baths. But one hears things."

"Such as?" I jingled the money-pouch in the pocket of my robe to let him know there was coin involved.

"Emil was, one might say, ambitious," Angie hedged. "He flaunted himself. He hinted at connections with the Upper Tier."

"Anything concrete?" I produced silver.

"It's possible the name Delrey came up," Angie said. "There have been sightings of certain members of that clan on Entertainment Row recently."

"I've seen Gorgeous Gyorgi and his playmates at Smokey Joe's," I mused. "Was Emil one of that lot?"

"Junior Banker Delrey has been seen in a number of inappropriate venues." Angie clearly didn't approve of the Upper Tier's forays into low life. "Emil was seen with him on occasion, but not as part of his, um, steady entourage. Emil preferred more stable patrons, older and wiser."

"The kind who pay well for their pleasures?"

Angie nodded gravely. "Emil made sure everyone knew just how expensive his, ah, company…was."

"Gorgeous Gyorgi's been throwing coin around," I pointed out.

"Junior Banker Delrey is totally dependent on his brother's good will. If Master Banker Vernor Delrey should cut off the funds, Junior Banker Delrey would not be so popular on Entertainment Row."

I summed it up. "So, Emil liked coin. Don't we all? He got it from senior males. No problem there— he was Licensed. Why the long face, Angie?'

"There are some senior males whose preferences are not well known, and who take steps to keep it that way. Emil was not as discreet as he should have been, particularly when discussing visitors to Lorr."

"'What happens in Lorr stays in Lorr'," I quoted the adage.

"Of course. It's why people come here," Angie said with a smirk. "For Rest and Recreation"

"Of the kind they can't find in Norland or Contramont." I didn't bother to mention South Coast. They've got Port Chicago, where they try to outdo Lorr in both entertainment and business. Let them try. Lorr has been around longer, and does it better.

"Mind you, I can't verify this," Angie said. "But I have heard that certain senior males were not above recommending Emil's services to their colleagues from other settlements."

"And Emil might have taken advantage of the opportunity to further his own interests?"

"Some of those visitors would be very unhappy if what happened in Lorr became known outside Lorr. Blackmail is such an unpleasant business. Even the Assassins look down on blackmailers."

"There are some things even the Fatsos won't touch," I agreed.

I wasn't going to get much more out of Angie. I handed him his coin, collected my cleaned clothes, and went back out onto Entertainment Row.

I chewed over the idea of Emil as a blackmailer. It was possible, but who was the target? Gorgeous Gyorgi made no secret of his taste for joyboys, so there was no point in blackmailing him. Zac was a student, no coin there.

There must be something else going on. As it stood now, Emil had been sent to seduce Zac and get the journal, then pass it on to the one who'd hired him. Instead, he'd decided to keep it for himself. Using it as a lever to pry more coin out of that someone? He should have known better than to provoke his clients. Desperate people did dangerous things.

Now I had to find out just who was that desperate.

ii

I stalked up and down Entertainment Row looking for joyboys. If they weren't out and about, the best place to find them was at the Green Dragon Casino and Cafe, opposite the Opera House.

The Opera House serves as a venue for spectacular performances in addition to the usual grand orchestral and musical events. It's also the unofficial headquarters for the Entertainment Guild. Sure, they have a Guild-hall on the Central Plaza, but that's where the contracts are signed and the records are kept. Legal stuff, handled by drones. The real business of Entertainment is conducted right there, on Entertainment Row, by the Representatives of the Guild.

Its top members keep their eyes open for new talent and regulate what does and does not get presented on stages and streets and taverns in Lorr, and by whom. It's no good trying to perform without paying the Entertainment Guild its fees. They'll find you and fine you, and you'll be back in the office or shop, or on the farm, slogging away without the applause or the coin. Even if the coin's not much, the applause makes up for it…or so they tell me. I prefer coin to applause.

The Upper Tier of the Entertainment Guild prefer to be called Impresarios or Representatives, depending on the specialty. The two theaters have their Reps—there's one for the buskers and another for the dancers. Female Licensees have people like Velda looking after their welfare. For male Licensees, the one in charge is Savvy Sal Flores.

Sal rose from being a joyboy himself to acting as Guild Rep for the male sex workers of Lorr. Sal knows everything about every male Licensee on Entertainment Row. If Emil was up to no good, Sal would have something to say about it.

I found him in his lair, a table in the open area of the Green Dragon between the gambling rooms and the eating establishment. The Dragon is a vast step up from Smokey Joe's, even though it serves the same function. The walls are covered with images of reptiles, real and imaginary, being slain by large, muscular males in minimal garb. The electrics were turned on, adding a garish glow to the painted spaces between images.

Sal Flores lounged at his table, surrounded by five of his favorite flunkies. They were a mixed lot—two in Pangkoti silk jackets and trou, one in Norland knitted tunic and woolly trou, two in Lorr's finest trou-and-jacket set, or an inexpensive approximation of the same. Not a multicolored kilt among them.

Sal is a fairskin with blue eyes, pale hair, and a wisp of something on his upper lip. Once muscular and trim, he's now running to fat around the middle. Today he was draped in a red silk robe embroidered with green and blue flowers, open to show the blue silk shirt and trou underneath. Very expensive, very showy, not a good choice for someone with his coloring, but who am I to criticize someone else's fashion sense?

"Oyo, Sal, how's business?" I greeted him. "Mind if I join you for a cup of chai?"

Sal sighed dramatically.

"Oyo, Drach. Business is dreadful, dreadful." He waved at the nearest server. "Chai for Eye Drach." He leaned forward, eyes glittering. "Did you hear what happened to Emil? Just dreadful."

"Not pleasant," I agreed. "Any ideas who might have done the deed?"

"They say he got on the wrong side of the Fatsos," one of the Lorran lads offered. "One of the new recruits. They seem to think they're still on Kunine's ship."

"They're getting far too aggressive," Sal added. "Fee M'Farr made a mistake taking them on."

"Could be Emil got in someone's way," I mused. "Visitors to Lorr sometimes get upset when they see male Licensees on the street."

The server set a small porcelain cup of chai in front of me. I sipped carefully, inhaling the fragrance. This was something to savor, well above the usual clet-stand sludge offered by most establishments on Entertainment Row.

"Emil wasn't on the stroll," the Norlander said. "He made a great point of it. He only worked the houses, or went to private homes, by appointment, for a very special clientele. Or so he said."

"Upper Tier, very exclusive," the Pangkoti added. "But not always. I saw him with a patron going into Vassily's Veranda not two days before it…happened."

Vassily's is one of the Accommodation Houses on Red Lantern Alley, rooms available for an hour or two. Useful for casual liaisons, mostly used by street Licensees or people who didn't want their doings noticed by spouses.

"A patron?" I digested this, along with the chai. "Upper Tier?"

"Not from Lorr. It looked like one of those characters from the Minerals." The Pangkoti tittered. "Beard, bibbed trou, straw hat. What would his mates think of him spending time with one of us?"

"Probably read him out of the Trade Delegation." Sal snickered.

"You think he was one of that lot?" I asked.

"Who else is in Lorr from Contramont? It's the wrong time of the year for the iron shipments."

That comment came from the Norlander—trust a Norland male to keep track of the ships going in and out of Lorr.

I considered this new evidence. "Could you recognize the visitor if you saw him again?"

The Pangkoti joyboy shook his head. "Not in front of a magistrate, I wouldn't. It was only in passing, and from a distance. All I saw was hat and beard, I couldn't say who was behind them."

"So, not a youngster? A grown male?"

"That far I'd go, but no further."

"It's enough to give me a few ideas," I said. "Here's something to buy clet."

The Pangkoti glanced at Sal, got a nod, and snatched up the coin.

Sal nodded to the entourage, who obediently moved to another table. "You didn't come here to drink chai," he said, leaning toward me. "What's the interest in Emil?"

"I've been hired to look into Emil's demise. There's something very dicey about it. I've heard some things about Emil."

"Such as?" Sal's eyes narrowed. "Rumors, gossip? Anything that's detrimental to the Guild, I want to know."

121

"It's been hinted that Emil used his contacts for personal gain beyond the usual fees, and didn't always report it to the Guild. That he might even have threatened to expose his activities with patrons to those who did not approve of them."

Now Sal was really interested. "Are you suggesting...blackmail?"

"Emil had a lot of coin," I said. "He passed it around. He was very generous to the soup-kitchens in Fishmarket, and wore fancy duds. He also dropped hints to his body-servant of a big score coming his way. I know he took something belonging to one of his clients, maybe at the request of another patron."

Sal's face grew redder with each word. "That is not Entertainment Guild policy," he sputtered. "Putting the black on a regular patron? Just not done! It's bad for business! And using what one learns in an intimate situation, that's worse."

"Oh, it gets better," I said. "It's just possible that one or the other of those patrons snuck into Emil's digs to stop him telling what he knew."

"That's not possible," Sal stated firmly. "How would he find out where Emil lived?"

"Emil had to go home sometime," I suggested. "He could even have brought the client with him."

"No one brings work home. That's what places like Vassily's Veranda are for. There has to be *some* privacy!"

"Well, someone must have found Emil's digs, because that's where he was..." I let it hang in the air. "There's a Fatso, a Pangkoti called Brutus—the Guards think he's the one, but I don't. If you hear anything, you can pass it on to Velda or Basher Bob at Smokey Joe's, and they'll get it to me."

I handed a silver to the server, waved to the joyboys, took my leave of the Green Dragon, and continued along Entertainment Row.

I was starting to build up a picture of Emil. A go-getter, a joyboy with ambitions. One who would do almost anything to get away from Entertainment Row, including blackmail.

One question remained: Who was the original intended extortion target? And how far were they ready to go to get rid of a leech?

I considered my next move. Smokey Joe's again? I decided against it. I needed rest, food that wasn't sludge, and a session with Ficus.

I threaded my way through the growing crowd of two-wheels and pedi-shaws and headed back to Foodie Alley. What I wanted was a quiet evening at home.

`I didn't get it.

iii

I was almost at Fletcher's when I heard a yell behind me.

"Pola Drach! Wait up!"

I turned around to see Basher Bob pounding through the crowd. He ran up to me, his face contorted with rage.

"Where've you been? I've been looking for you all over the place."

"You didn't look in the baths. What's got your trou in a twist?"

"The futtering Guards have picked up Brutus."

"Already? That was fast. They only found the body this afternoon."

"Which body is this? The one they picked Brutus up for was Emil," Basher clarified "He's charged with Unsanctioned Killing."

"Not the student at the Academy?"

"Not that I heard. What is this about a student?"

"That Contramonter we sent on his way. He never made it back to his lodgings, wound up at the bottom of the cliff, in a patch of vampire vines. When was this arrest?"

"About an hour ago. A squad picked him up at his doss. One of the Pangkoti hardbodies came to Smokey Joe's to tell me. According to him, they took Brutus off to Admin Detention in a skimmer."

I took a minute to think it over. "That's just not right," I said. "Who ordered the arrest?"

"My pals at the Waterfront Guardhouse saw Captain Atterson overseeing the Special Squad."

"Death and Destruction!" I swore. "Are you sure the charge was for Emil's murder? Not the student?"

"According to what Brutus's friend heard. Where does the Conty come in?"

"It was his book Emil was supposed to hand over to Brutus, but Brutus swears by all the gods of Pangkot he never got it. As for Zac, I talked to Brutus this morning, and he told me he left the lad at the Advanced Academy carrier station, then went back to his own doss. No reason for him to lie."

"And you say the lad is dead?"

"He wound up in a patch of vampire vines. I don't know if he was alive when the vines got to him, but he wasn't by the time he was hauled out."

Basher dragged me out of the crowd into the space between two clet-stands.

"Atterson never charged him with the student, but he's going down for Emil. There's at least two witnesses who saw him coming out of the joyboys' lodgings. What do you think we should do? He's your client as well as mine; we both took his coin."

I looked around. We were a few steps from Fletcher's Food Shop. The place was almost empty, no one there but Fletcher. I led Basher into the shop, sat at my favorite table in the corner, and yelled,"Chai! And clet!" I wasn't about to get muzzy on brew, not with everything going down at once.

Fletcher hustled up the drinks, dropped them on the table, and retreated to his kitchen.

I took a swig of chai. It wasn't anything as nice as what I'd had at the Green Dragon.

"Let the Fatsos deal with it," was my first response to Basher, "Brutus signed on with the Assassins' Guild. That's why we have Guilds in the first place, so they can take care of their own."

"I don't see Fee M'Farr moving too fast on this," Basher said. "No coin for him, and Brutus isn't really one of his own, not even one of his better Fatsos. He's new, and he's Pangkoti. He'll be hung out to dry, like washing on the line."

"And you'll be out one client," I observed. "But as I see it, M'Farr is caught between two poles. He's got to keep his Fatsos in line, can't let them take extra work, especially not Unsanctioned Killings. At the same time, he's got to back his people up when they get into trouble. At least provide an advocate. If Brutus gets a raw deal, it's no fault of yours, and no breach of contract."

"It's not that. It's...it's unfair, is what it is. Brutus is being targeted just because it's convenient. Atterson needs to find someone to arrest, Brutus was spotted at the scene, and that's enough for a magistrate to send him off to the mines for a winter or two."

I shrugged. "He looks tough enough to stand a little cold weather, and hard work never hurt anyone."

Basher took a pull at his clet. "It's still not right."

"What's it to you?"

He looked into his mug. "I've been there. I don't want a client of mine sent to the mines, even a lowlife like Brutus."

I had to agree. "Brutus isn't my favorite person. He's a rapist, and probably a killer, but he's not the one who did Emil in. If he goes down for this, there'll someone out there feeling very smug because he got away with murder. Twice," I added. "I saw a red line on Boffin Zac's throat when they hauled him out of the vampire vines. Someone took a cord to him, just like with Emil. Two murders, same killer."

Basher made a noise of disgust. "If his Guild won't help him..." He looked at me with pleading eyes. "You've got the connections, Pola. And he's partly your client, too."

"What you mean is, you want me to go over to the Central Guardhouse and see Brutus. Find out exactly what happened, get him out of detention. He's your client, Basher. I'm just a side player in this kickball game."

"I don't like Admin. Never did." Basher's soulful eyes looked into mine. "But you're their kind, you can talk to them. Find out things I can't. I can go up and down the Waterfront and talk to the rest of Kunine's people, check out Brutus's story, while you deal with the Upper Tier."

"You're right. I can deal with Admin." I grew up with the Upper Tier. I understand how they operate. They spend their entire lives playing elaborate lizard-against-rodent games, everyone looking for an edge in an endless contest for dominance.

That's why I deal mostly with the Middle Tier. I let Basher handle the hardbodies and lowlifes while I cope with the office drones. Let the Brain match wits with the Uppers. I stay out of it.

"You go to Admin," Basher continued. "Find out what you can, then go over to Arriver's Hill and find an advocate to take on Brutus's case. I'll see if I can find someone who'll testify that Brutus wasn't anywhere near Emil when it happened. Send word to Velda at Smokey Joe's when you have more info."

"One more thing," I said. "Find that street lizard, Jakki, and keep him safe. If nothing else, *he* can get Brutus out of detention. Jakki saw Emil on the floor long before Brutus even got there. If the killer gets wind of a witness…" I didn't have to finish.

Basher nodded. "There's always a gang of street lizards hanging around the Drushka Vikk-shop—I think they're Jakki's friends. They might know where he is. When I find him, I'll get Velda to keep him under wraps. You go over to the Central Guardhouse, talk to Atterson, get Brutus out of there."

For a moment, I considered running upstairs to give Ficus a quick spritz and a spoonful of clet. Then I decided I'd have plenty of time once I finished with Brutus. Humans come before plants, and business comes before everything in Lorr.

I spotted a free pedi-shaw and decided to treat myself to a decent ride. I hopped on, waved goodbye to Basher, and settled onto the seat. Things were moving too fast; someone was pulling strings. There were too many threads to this tangled web—nothing made sense.

iv

I was still mulling over things when the pedi-shaw pulled up at the plaza in front of the Central Guardhouse. The late-afternoon sun cast long shadows across the open space. The food vendors were packing up their carts, marking the end of the working day. Guards streamed in and out of the building, changing shifts.

Getting to see someone like Captain Sara Atterson wasn't as easy as just walking in and asking politely. I had to run the usual gauntlet of underlings and pass a coin or two before I was let into her lair.

It was a different office from her previous post—a square cell in the middle of the Guardhouse hive. Not much larger than my own office, but bigger than her last one, furnished with the usual desk, two chairs, and file shelves. Its only virtue was privacy.

Seated at her desk, Atterson didn't bother to stand to greet me. She looked up from a pile of papers and growled, "Independent Eye Drach. I suppose you're here to collect."

"Collect what?" I hadn't expected that.

"Reward offered for information leading to the arrest of one Assassin called Brutus." She indicated the other chair, an offer to sit down. I took it.

"I heard he was taken in. On what evidence?"

"He was seen going into Emil's rooms and coming out again. The Medical Examiner found his fingerprints all over the room. You told me yourself he'd accompanied the student on the carrier. He was present at both murders, so he's the most likely to have done it."

"Sure, he was there, at Emil's. He told me so himself."

"Oh?" Atterson put a wealth of meaning into one syllable. "I didn't know you were that cozy with Pangkoti Assassins."

"He's Basher Bob's client, not mine, but Basher asked me to put in a good word for him."

"Let him come here himself."

"Basher doesn't like the City Guards," I explained. "As for Brutus, I don't know what the medical report says, but according to what Dark One Kelvin told me, Emil had been gone for at least twelve hours before your lot got there. I've got a witness who will testify he saw

Emil on the floor while it was still dark. Brutus didn't go into the house until after daybreak, and Emil was finished well before then. What else have you got?"

"Seems Friend Brutus and Joyboy Emil were seen several times together. The last time was the day Emil met his end. The two were not on good terms."

"That doesn't mean Brutus took a cord to Emil's throat," I pointed out. "He'd be more likely to use a knife in an argument. As for his whereabouts on the night in question, you can check his sign-ins. The Flatlands Force checks in and out with the City Guards at the bridge."

"I can do that. It'll take some time, though. Meanwhile, Brutus stays in custody."

"Where's he now?"

"In the holding area, pending removal to Admin Security. We're taking no chances with this one."

"Has he contacted his Guild?" According to the Regs of Lorr, anyone accused of a crime should have legal advice provided, either by the appropriate Guild or by Admin.

"He sent a message to Master Assassin M'Farr," Atterson admitted. "I don't know if M'Farr cares enough to come himself, or if he'll send one of his flunkies."

"Can I see him?"

"What for? You say he's not your client, he's Bob's. What's your interest in this Pangkoti pirate?"

"There's something wrong about this whole setup," I said. "It's not like I care all that much for Brutus. He was one of Ishka Kunine's lot, no doubt about it. He was involved in the attack on Merchant Beatriz Vikk.

He may have been one of the hardbodies who menaced shopkeepers, forced them to sell bad merch. He even took a swing at me a time or two.

"But he didn't do Emil in, and he definitely didn't do the boffin on the beach. I can't let him go down for either of those two. Nail him on something else, but not the joyboy and not the boffin."

"If you mean the Contramonter, he's been cleared of that one. It's been declared an unfortunate accident," Atterson said slowly. "The poor sod must have mistaken his way and fallen over the railing, into the vampire vines."

"And the mark around his throat?" I was sure I'd seen one.

"His shirt-string must have got caught in the railing. Leave this one alone, Drach." Her voice held a note of warning. "I've been told, and I'm telling you. It was an accident, and nothing else."

"I can't leave it alone. I know what I saw. Brutus didn't do the deed on Zac, but someone did. Someone's pulled an Unsanctioned Killing, and when M'Farr finds out, he's going to be furious. I may have another client on my hands."

Atterson shrugged, then fished a token off her desk. "What you do with Master Assassin M'Farr is your business. Here's a pass, go see your client. Maybe you'll change your mind when you talk with him."

I accepted the token that would get me into the holding area. "By the way, who posted the reward?"

"Reward is in care of the Delrey Bank," Atterson said, with a smirk. "Seems someone in the Delrey household is really upset about Emil. That joyboy must have meant a lot to that someone."

"Indeed, he must have." I rose and headed for the holding area. One more thread in the tangle!

v

The holding pen in the Central Guardhouse is at the back of the basement, well below street level in what must have been the Founders' bunker many generations ago. It hasn't improved with age. It's cold, dank, and dark, with electrics providing light and a wheezy system blowing air through the corridors.

A disgruntled male guard led me through the maze of corridors to a bare room with a table, two chairs, and a mirror on one wall, obviously a spy portal. Another guard led Brutus in.

"No funny stuff," he warned. He stood at the door, hand on his bludgeon, to make sure.

"He won't pull anything," I assured him. "Will you?"

Brutus grumbled something in Pangkoti. The guard stepped away, leaving me to deal with Brutus on my own. I had no doubt there would be someone on the other side of the wall watching and listening.

"I'm no advocate, I don't expect privacy." I nodded toward the mirror. "If you've got anything else to say, now's the time to say it."

Brutus frowned. "I can't tell you any more than I already did. It's like I told those Guards. I came off shift, I saw a fella, he told me to get the book from Emil, and gave me coin to do it. When I went into Emil's room, I saw him on the floor. I got out, fast."

"But not before you searched the place," I reminded him. "That you didn't tell me. The Dark Ones found your foot and fingerprints all over the room."

"Can they really do that?"

"You'd be surprised what the Dark Ones can find, given enough time. Let's go over it again. You got off shift and passed the guards at the bridge?"

Brutus nodded. "That's what I said."

"And someone called to you?"

"Like I said."

"How did he call? What did he say? Was it, 'You, Flatlands Force'? Or, 'Oyo, Pangkoti pirate'?"

Brutus thought a bit. "He called me by name," he said. "He called out 'Brutus', and I went over to the Guardhouse, and there was someone in the shadows."

"Try to remember what he looked like. You said it was a male?"

"Unless there's a female my size, maybe even taller. And the voice was low, and sort of, you know, hifalutin'. Kinda like Banker Selva Delrey."

"You say this fella knew you by name?" I considered that bit of information. "How so? You've only been in Lorr since Ishka Kunine landed, before summer. He took off two double-moons ago."

"Left us flat, he did!" Brutus burst out. "Me and Casem and Kayto and the rest, anyone who was ashore. He just sailed off and left us here to fend for ourselves!" He seemed justly affronted by such disloyalty. Captains aren't supposed to desert their crews.

"I suppose he thought he'd pick you up when he came back in triumph," I said. "Only that didn't happen. So, you took what you could get and signed up with the Fatsos."

"The Honorable Guild of Forgers, Assassins, Thieves, and Swindlers," Brutus said with some pride. "I paid my entrance fee, I got the sigil, and the assurance from Master Assassin Fee M'Farr himself that I'd be taken care of."

"Unless you broke faith with him," I reminded him. "Master Assassin M'Farr doesn't take kindly to those who break Guild rules. If he thinks you took coin for a private job and didn't pass it along to the Guild, he'll turn you over to Admin without mussing a hair on his head."

Brutus grabbed my hand. "Eye Drach, you have the Master Assassin's ear. Tell him I didn't do Emil!"

I pulled away. "I'm convinced you didn't kill that joyboy. In fact, I'm beginning to have a notion as to who did. But there's no proof, and right now, you're the only one who even looks like a suspect."

"I swear by Mata Diva…"

"Does no good in Lorr. We don't bother with sworn oaths. Evidence, that's what's needed. So…back to your story. You think the person who paid you to get the book from Emil knew you?"

"I guess he must have," Brutus said.

"How many people in Lorr know you by that name?"

Brutus's brow wrinkled in thought. "Not that many. I've got my own mates, and there's the Flatlands Force, and some of the folks at Smokey Joe's. And you, and Bob, and M'Farr, and the Delreys…" His voice trailed off as he realized what he'd said. "Mata Diva protect me! It couldn't have been someone who knew me from Banker Selva's boat, could it? She had some mechs, borrowed from her brother's crew. It could have been one of them."

"It seems you have some powerful friends...or enemies," I said. "And just how well did you know Emil? According to Captain Atterson, there are witnesses who say you had words on the day he met his end."

Brutus shifted in his chair. "That was personal."

"How personal?" I persisted.

"It was about the lad...Jakki. I didn't like the way he was being treated."

"Jakki seems to have thought the world of Emil. He even came to me, asked me to find out who did him in if it wasn't you."

"Maybe, but I still didn't like it. Those lads, they'll cozy up to anyone who feeds them, gives them a doss. I saw how Emil ordered Jakki around, made him wait up till all hours, had him running his errands, carrying his messages. The lad deserved better."

"And you would have given it to him?"

"I would have, if Emil was willing to let him go. I told him so one time when I saw him at puja. He got all huffy and said it was Jakki's decision to stick with him and none of my business. What he and Jakki did or didn't do, I should keep my nose out of it."

I wanted to get more out of him, but the guard at the door banged on the wall.

"Time's up!" He leered at Brutus. "You're a popular fella, Pangkoti. There's someone else to see you."

Brutus perked up. "Master Assassin M'Farr?"

"Himself. You must have done something really big to get all this attention."

"I didn't kill that joyboy!"

I got up from my seat. "I'll try to get Atterson to see reason. Right now, you have to make it good with your Guild. Tell M'Farr what you told me, let him deal with Admin—it's what the Guildmaster does."

I had one more fact to go on—Brutus's connection with the Delrey clan. I had no idea why, or how, but I was sure of one thing. The Delrey bankers were at the bottom of this murky mess. All I had to do was prove it.

vi

I met Fee M'Farr in the corridor and blocked him before he went into the interrogation room. He looked less like a grocer and more like an assassin today, stout in a well-cut jacket and trou, flanked by Ratty on one side and Cahane Roy, his personal advocate, on the other.

"Oyo, Master Assassin," I greeted him. "How's business?"

He didn't bother with manners. "What's this deathly excrement about one of my men being involved in an Unsanctioned Killing?"

"That's what he's charged with. He swears by the Pangkoti deity he didn't do it, and I believe him."

"And I should believe you?" M'Farr sneered.

"I don't lie, especially not to you. I've never steered you wrong, Master Assassin. There's someone in Lorr who did this, but it's not Brutus."

136

"He took coin," M'Farr groused. "and didn't report it. That's against Guild policy."

"Not for killing anyone," I pointed out. "It was for a simple errand. Give the male a break. He hasn't had time to get to the baths, let alone the Guild. He'd have shared, sooner or later. And according to him, it wasn't all that much, anyway."

"The exact sum doesn't matter. He didn't report it. I can't let that go by. Discipline must be maintained." He started toward the interrogation room. I stepped in front of him again.

"Master Assassin, I don't want to tell you how to conduct your business…"

"Isn't that what you're doing?" He shoved me aside.

"I just want to point out that your hold on the Guild depends on the loyalty of your people. This Pangkoti, Brutus, was one of the new hires, the ones you personally approved. If you don't back him when he's down, the rest of the Pangkoti will take it as a sign that your word is no good. "

M'Farr stopped in mid-stride. "No one says that!"

"Master Assassin, you trusted me once to get information you needed. Trust me again. Give me a day, and I'll have some answers."

He thought it over. "I'll have a word with Friend Brutus. He'll get the best advocate I've got. But he's got to be straight with me, or I'll hand him to Admin to send to the mines."

"I think someone's playing a deep game," I said. "And we're just pieces on the gameboard. But he's just made a bad mistake, and I can use that to untangle this mess. Give me the time, and I'll do it. Not for you, and not for Brutus, but for me, and for Lorr."

M'Farr nodded, then went into the interrogation room. That left it to me to find my way out of the labyrinth back to the fading daylight of the plaza.

I chewed over what I had learned, what had been said, and what hadn't been said. I was jolted out of my thoughts by someone yelling at me.

"Oyo! Drach!"

It was Reg Bonwit, with a pedi-shaw.

"Hop in, Pola. The Brain wants to see you."

BRAIN POWER

I DIDN'T HAVE MUCH CHOICE. WHEN JULIAN HUNT wants to see you, you go.

Julian Hunt is something of an institution in Lorr. She's been resident in the house on Arriver's Hill since before the Merchant's War. Before that, rumor is she was a top boffin at the Advanced Academy. Or maybe one of the major players in Admin Security. Or else she was involved in some heavy dealings between the former Autocrat of Pangkot and the Admin Executive.

No one knows for sure, and no one is about to try to find out.

What is definitely known about Julian Hunt is that she never leaves the house on Arriver's Hill, that she's an expert on the native plants of New Earth, and that she's the one the Upper Tier goes to when they get into a mess they don't want to hand to the City Guards or their Guild Security.

She's also the one I went to after I was asked to leave the Guards. I lasted about a week—I couldn't deal with her moods and constant orders. She sent me on my way with a seedling called Ficus and took on Reg instead.

How he manages to get along with her I'll never understand, but he's been doing it for years. Reg Bonwit is her right hand. Also her legs, eyes, and ears. He runs around Lorr getting information for her to digest along with super-lush meals she concocts with her personal cook, Freddy Burns.

Julian Hunt, Basher Bob, and I are the only Independent Eyes in Lorr. There are plenty of other investigators, all spying on each other, reporting to their Guilds. We three are the only ones not connected with any particular Guild, or with Administration, or the Dark Ones, or the Advanced Academy. We don't owe anything to anyone except our clients—Upper, Lower, or Middle Tier. Humans are humans, no matter what their status, and everyone needs help at one time or another. We provide the answers to their questions, offer solutions to their problems. What do they do next? That's up to the client.

I hopped into the pedi-shaw alongside Reg.

"What's up?" I asked as the driver threaded his way down the Grand Boulevard through the late-day traffic. The sun was down, the two moons weren't going to show on a moondark night, and the electrics threw shadows across the crowd of office drones and shop clerks going back to Flatlands for their evening meal. A sharp breeze rustled in the gaps between shops, sending dry leaves and dust whirling in the air. Winter was on its way for sure.

"I gave that book to Eye Hunt," Reg said.

"I hope she appreciated the gesture."

"She had a look at it." Reg wasn't giving anything away. "But before she could do anything about it, she got a visit from the Contramont Miners Trade Delegation, howling for action."

"Without an appointment? And you let them in?"

"They're clients."

That explained everything. Julian Hunt charges ten times what I do, but her clients can afford it. It all goes to the upkeep of that house and its precious greenhouse of rare plants. She may be top tier, but she still has to fulfill her contractual obligations.

"What did they want?"

"Elder Pinkney isn't satisfied that poor Zac went over the railing on his own, and wants Hunt to look into it. He's convinced it has something to do with the missing funds."

"How so?"

"He had a conversation with the lad after their weekly prayer meeting last week. The lad was troubled, said he'd seen and heard something that worried him, and didn't know what to do about it. Elder Pinkney asked why he didn't take his troubles to his sponsor, and the lad said it was Elder Mackintosh he'd seen, in conversation with someone in Delrey livery."

That sounded very familiar. I'd once been in a similar position. I reported what I'd seen and heard, and paid for it by being asked to leave the Guards. I wound up living over Fletcher's, taking a room behind Jake and Holly's, and setting up as an Independent Eye. Apparently, what Zac had seen carried worse consequences.

"And then…?"

"Pinkney went to Mackintosh, who seems to have calmed Pinkney's jitters, but the Contramonter's doubts are growing. He's convinced someone from the Delreys got to someone in the Contramont Delegation, and he wants Hunt to do more digging."

"And Eye Hunt's opinion?"

"I told her what had happened at the recycling beach, and what you and I saw. Then I gave her the book. She was intrigued enough to send me out to track you down. Now, you tell me, what's this guff about Fatso Brutus doing in Licensee Emil?"

"Guff is what it is," I agreed. "Captain Atterson's being pushed to close the case, and she's lit on the likeliest suspect. She's wrong, but I can't prove it without Jakki, and that street lizard's making himself scarce. He popped up long enough to give me the book, then took off before I could stop him. Probably found a hidey-hole somewhere in Fishmarket with the rest of his friends."

"Probably a good idea. Sounds like someone's tying up loose ends."

We'd reached Arriver's Hill. Reg helped me down from the pedi-shaw, paid off the driver, and started for the door to Hunt's house just as four males decked out in Contramont gear emerged.

I pulled him back into the shadow of the building so we couldn't be seen.

"Is that...?"

"Contramont Miner's Trade Delegation," Reg hissed at me. "I thought they'd left."

"Or maybe they came back," I said. "Who's who? I know Mackintosh—he gave his name when we met in front of the Temple of Healing. But who are the others? They didn't introduce themselves then."

"The short one with the gray beard is Elder Pinkney. The long noodle in the middle is Elder Kennington. The two of them were sent all the way from Contramont to oversee the negotiations.

"The big youngster is one of their so-called attendants. Bodyguards, more likely. They came with the Elders to protect them from big, bad Lorr." Reg snickered. "There are some more stout lads hanging around the house in Garden Sector, miners from the look of them."

"I thought Mackintosh was in charge of the negotiations?"

"Not according to Pinkney and Kennington. Mackintosh is the liaison, not the final signer. They're the ones with the authority to conclude the deal."

The group conferred loudly on the street in front of the house. Once you got past the Conty twang, the quarrel was easy to overhear. They didn't seem to know or care whether anyone was listening.

"I told you to let me handle things," Mackintosh spat. "Master Banker Delrey was ready to sign the contracts. We could have finished this whole business, and you could be back on the transport before the winter storms make it impossible to travel."

"Master Banker Delrey's terms are unacceptable," Pinkney retorted. "And we cannot go back home until we find out how our dear brother Zacharias met his end."

"And what happened to our funds." That was Kennington, in a nasal Conty twang. "I do not understand why you insisted on consulting this person, Hunt. Why not use the services of one of the Guilds with whom we have had dealing? And why didn't you warn us this so-called Independent Eye was a woman?"

"You were the one who insisted on consulting someone not connected with the Construction Guild or the Administration. Independent Eye Hunt is known to most of the Upper Tier of Lorr," Mackintosh protested. "My contacts at the Construction and Transport guilds tell me she conducts her investigations with discretion and dispatch.

"And as for my work…" He sounded positively affronted. "I have been negotiating for the Contramont Miners for nearly twenty years, not only in Lorr but in Pangkot and South Coast. I have never had my integrity questioned before."

"I still don't see why we couldn't rely on the Construction Guild Security Force to find out what happened to poor Zac," Kennington complained.

"I do not think Construction Guild agents have the knowledge necessary to uncover the truth behind the demise of our young brother." Pinkney tried to soothe his ruffled companion. "One of our brightest boffins, cut off in his prime! One who was behind a major advance in our technology, who had devised a method for extracting more energy from our product.

"Clearly, Brother Mackintosh, someone must have wanted him removed before he could announce his findings, patent his apparatus, and allow us to benefit from his discoveries."

Mackintosh stared his shorter colleague down. "I have the report from the Dark Ones. It has been determined that Brother Zacharias met with a dreadful accident," he stated. "Bad enough that we have to bring the inner workings of the Contramont Miners Trade Delegation under scrutiny. There was no need for you to drag Eye Hunt into looking for any other cause for his death. As for the other matter, I'm sure she will agree there is no malfeasance here, only some small errors in accounting."

"And what about the deficiency of funds? The unpaid bills? The shipments gone astray? Those, Brother Mackintosh, are far more important issues than the demise of a foolish lad." Elder Kennington turned on Mackintosh. "Brother Zacharias was insistent that he saw you in conversation with one of the Delrey mechanicals."

"That may well be, but it was quite innocent, I assure you. Master Banker Delrey has been most helpful in settling the terms of our agreement. What Brother Zacharias saw was an exchange of messages regarding meeting times, no more."

"Banker Delrey is attempting to reword our contracts to his own advantage!" Kennington countered. "And he is tempting our people with pleasures. I fear you have become corrupted by the fleshpots of this sinful place, Brother. You even encouraged our young people to attend that disgusting revelry in Red Lantern Alley.

"Oh, yes, I know all about it, how they were plied with alcohol and with female company, all to coax our trade secrets and production methods from us."

"You are too hard on Banker Delrey." Mackintosh joined Pinkney in trying to calm Kennington. "Let us go back to the residence and have dinner. You will feel better once you're fed."

They headed down the hill to the Grand Boulevard, where they found transportation back to their lodgings.

Reg and I looked at each other in disbelief.

"Disharmony among the Contys. Will wonders never cease," I said.

"Come on in, Pola. The Brain awaits.

ii

The sight of Julian Hunt in full bloom was enough to take my breath away. To say she's large is like saying the ocean is wet, or the Mineral Mountains are high.

She's taller and broader than a lot of males, and tends to drape herself in caftans, in the wildly colored patterns popular just before the Merchant's War, with a matching head-wrap. That day, the caftan was bright orange, with green and purple spots. Her head was wrapped in a purple scarf. She had pink facepaint on her lips and cheeks and bright blue on her eyelids.

She sat behind a massive desk as Reg let me into her inner chamber—the library where she spends her time when she isn't in the rooftop greenhouse or the basement kitchen.

She greeted us with a wave of the hand. "Independent Eye Pola Drach. It's been some time."

"Independent Eye Julian Hunt." I nodded. "I'm always ready to assist when called on. I am in your debt, especially for Ficus. The last time was two years ago. I hope I provided the information you needed?"

"I have no complaints. The witness you discovered helped to convict a financial fraudster."

That one had not been a registered member of the Honorable Guild of Forgers, Assassins, Thieves, and Swindlers, but an outsider from South Coast, peddling fake shares in a nonexistent business enterprise. Fee M'Farr was furious with him, had him prosecuted and sent for a long stretch in the mines, mostly because none of his people had thought of doing it first.

"Do you need my services again?" I wished she'd get on with it. My stomach was reminding me it hadn't been filled all day with anything but chai, and I'd emptied that at the sorting beach. I wanted to get back to Fletcher's for my usual meal of roast beast and root-veg, and I had a twinge of guilt about leaving Ficus alone for so long..

"I've something else in mind." She rose. "Have you dined?"

"Not recently," I admitted.

"You will join me."

She swept ahead of me across the hall to the dining room, with Reg behind me. Probably to make sure I didn't escape. There wasn't much use in trying, anyway. I was doomed to eat whatever her cook set before us.

Dining with Julian Hunt was an adventure, one I tried hard to avoid whenever possible. I usually eat what I can afford, without much thought as to its origin or its flavor. If it doesn't poison me, I ingest it. How it is cooked, where it comes from, I really don't want to know. Most citizens of Lorr feel the same. Veg-sauce covers a lot of culinary sins.

Julian Hunt is one of the major exceptions to that way of thinking and eating. She is a vocal promoter of

the Healthy Food Movement, blasting the use of pro-
cessed foods and encouraging small shopkeepers to grow
their own vegetables. She has protested imports from
Pangkot as being unfit for consumption. She backs the
Dark Ones' constant monitoring of the fish coming into
the market. She praises Norlanders for coming up with
new uses for native herbs and tubers .She writes articles,
published in *Life-Style Mag*. In short, she's a food fanatic, which I most definitely am not.

Having one room designated solely for eating is an
extravagance in Lorr, where every inch of space is valuable. Most houses have a food-prep area with a table and
chairs where people can sit and eat what's been cooked,
without much ceremony. Julian Hunt's dining room is
dominated by a large round table set with pottery plat-
ters and glass receptacles for liquids. The usual eating
tools were placed on either side of the plates. In other
words, Upper Tier, as depicted in mags, based on tales
of Old Earth.

I noted the three settings. "You knew I was coming?"

Hunt took her seat and motioned for Reg to sit at
her right, me at her left.

"I thought you might need sustenance. Reg told
me how you reacted to the...the discovery. We will discuss that later. I do not wish to talk about business while
I dine."

What she did talk about, at length, was the geology
of New Earth, as evidenced by discoveries in Norland,
published in a recent mag, and backed by boffins sent
to track down the origins of reptiles. While she told me

more about fossils in rocks than I ever wanted to know, I dealt with the meal.

It began with a bowl of soup, brown and rich, but so spicy I could hardly get it over my tongue. Then, a bowl of mixed raw greens topped with something vinegary. Then a slab of fish covered in a pink sauce, also spicy, and served with more veg—steamed, not stewed, and crispy.

We ended with a large bowl of chopped-up fruit covered with sweet cream, something I haven't seen since my enforced sojourn in Norland some fifteen years ago. Cheese can withstand the perils of transport; liquids don't make it to the table quite as easily. The only mammals close to Lorr are goats, and I've never been fond of goat's milk.

I got through dinner by resorting to the liquid in the glass vessels, something fruity with a little tang to it. It tasted familiar, and it cut the spice somewhat.

"Norland cider," Reg tried to warn me. "Don't drink too much of it."

I should have listened.

By the end of the meal, my tongue and my brain were feeling fatigued. I was ready to head back to my cosy room and Ficus.

I didn't reckon with Julian Hunt.

"We may now proceed," she decreed.

Which we did, back to the library, where a surprise waited.

"Basher?" I certainly wouldn't have expected to see him in Hunt's orbit, let alone her library.

He got up from the chair where he'd been stationed, showing he was dressed in his best lizard leathers—matching trou and jacket—and a neck scarf, a sure sign he was in the presence of Upper Tier.

"I got your message. What's up?"

iii

Hunt took her place behind the desk, with Reg in a nearby chair. Basher sat back in the big red padded chair directly in front of the desk. I took a smaller chair with a yellow seat-pad and waited for the Brain to tell us why she'd summoned us to her sanctum.

"I have been considering the events of the last few days," she began. "Eye Bonwit has informed me that you, Eye Basheer, are looking into the accusations against the male called Brutus, formerly a member of Captain Ishka Kunine's crew, now employed by the Guild of Forgers, Assassins, Thieves, and Swindlers as part of their so-called Flatlands Force."

"That's right," Basher said. "And it's a crock. I've heard his story, and so has Pola. He says he didn't kill that joyboy, and I believe him."

"Do you, Eye Drach?" She turned her head towards me.

"I do. The timing's wrong. He says he saw the body on the floor when he went in. That means after sun-up, and Emil was gone long before then. At least, that's what the Dark One who investigated says, and he's one of the best."

"The whole thing sounds like something out of one of those story mags," Basher said. "Too complicated for someone like Brutus to come up with. Some male calls to him from the shadows, tells him to get a book from Joyboy Emil and bring it to the Guardhouse at the bridge, gives him a bag of coin and vanishes into the fog."

"Hmph!" Hunt made a noise of total disbelief.

"So, I checked it out. Sure thing, I found one of the Guards who remembers a male telling them that if a certain package arrives, they're to hold it until it's picked up. And a generous donation came with the instructions."

"I don't suppose they could identify this generous donor?" Reg had to put in his two coppers.

"The Guard was being cagey, but did say the donor left in a private pedi-shaw with the Delrey Bank sigil on the back panel."

Hunt turned back to me. "You were hired to retrieve a book, were you not, Eye Drach?"

"By a young Contramont boffin, Zac Garber," I said. "He'd been set up at some kind of party, more of an orgy, at Pegeen's Pleasure Palace, where he had an, um, encounter with Friend Emil. The book went missing right after that, so he thought it might have been lost at the Pleasure Palace."

"This book." Hunt withdrew it from somewhere under the desk.

"That's the one. Leather binding, handwritten. Boffin Zac called it his journal, said it contained his work and his private thoughts. I can't read it, it's in some kind of personal code."

"Not a code—an antiquated lettering system," Hunt corrected me. "I have not had time to examine it more thoroughly, because I was interrupted by the Contramont Miners' Trade Delegation."

She glared at Reg, who looked embarrassed.

"I didn't know they'd come without warning," he apologized. "I told them you'd send for them when you had more information. They didn't believe me, insisted on waiting until you got out of your plant rooms. I hoped they'd get tired of waiting and leave. Pola and I saw them outside. They weren't happy."

"There was some disagreement, but two of them were really upset at what happened to young Zac," I put in. "And I don't blame them. It was awful. Vampire vines kill slowly."

"Unless he was gone before he went over the railing," Reg said. "And if you're right, he was garroted before he went over."

Hunt summed it up. "It is clear we are all investigating aspects of the same set of circumstances. Eye Basheer's client Brutus is accused of removing Licensee Emil, who may have stolen the book Eye Drach's client lost, while my clients are demanding that I find the one who killed their young boffin. It would be to all our benefits if we work together to determine who is behind these events."

As always, Basher got to the heart of the matter. "Who pays? I don't know about you two, but I'm in this for the coin."

"You and Eye Drach have already taken fees for your work," Hunt said. "I will pay for any extraneous expenses you may incur."

Between the Brain's fluting voice, the weird food, the Norland cider, and sheer fatigue, my head was beginning to swim; but I retained enough sense to ask the next, obvious question.

"Where do we go from here?"

The Brain thought for all of two seconds.

"Eye Basheer, you have a female companion?"

"Velda, sure."

"Between the two of you, you can find out more about that party at the Pleasure Palace. Who set it up, who attended it, how it ended."

"How it ended? With a squad of City Guards called to stop a gang of Pangkoti hardbodies from wiping the floor with the Contys." Basher guffawed. "A bunch of so-called bodyguards. Never fought anything stronger than a large lizard."

"That, too, is suspicious," Hunt pointed out. "Report back here tomorrow. I am sure you will discover exactly who organized this spree, and who was involved in it."

"Can do." Basher grinned.

"Eye Drach!"

I sat up quickly. I was nearly dozing off in that chair.

"Tomorrow, go to the Advanced Academy Stranger's Hostel. Find out as much as you can about this young boffin. Who was he? Did he have any friends, any intimate companions? Had he made enemies?"

Exactly what I'd been planning to do anyway. I nodded, unable to speak coherently.

"What about *him*?" Basher glowered at Reg.

"Eye Bonwit will visit the residence in Garden Sector currently occupied by the Contramont Miner's Trade Delegation and obtain more information about their doings. What the difficulty is in the negotiations, who the principals are. And most specifically, who attended that gathering at the Pleasure Palace, and what took place there."

Basher didn't look happy about our assignments. "And what are you going to do while we're running around Lorr?"

"I shall endeavor to make sense of these adolescent maunderings. Good evening, Eye Basheer, Eye Drach. I suggest you take a pedi-shaw. It is a long way back to your lodgings."

She picked up the book. We had been dismissed.

Basher and I followed Reg down the hill to the Grand Boulevard. Luck was with us, and we found what must have been the last pedi-shaw on the route for the night.

"Get her home!" Reg ordered the driver.

I guess he did. I woke up in my own bed the next morning, more or less clothed, with a pounding head and roiling tum.

iv

I will never drink that Norland cider again. It's worse than jack. At least with jack the taste is enough to warn you what's coming at you. I'll stick to chai and brew from now on.

I managed to get out of my soiled clothes and into a new outfit, from the underpinnings out. Blue jacket with reversible lining, blue trou, pink shirt, workable walking boots. I sluiced off my face, took care of the teeth, and arranged my hair in a quick twist at the back of my neck.

I apologized profusely to Ficus for having left it alone for so long. I watered it, spritzed it with the special spray, spooned extra bonemeal and clet powder into its pot. I gave it an extra rub, checked carefully under each leaf for mites or other creepy-crawlies that might have blown in while I was out. I put it in a nice position a little ways back from the window, where it could get plenty of light but wouldn't be in a draft. I told it I'd be back before nightfall, and really hoped that was true.

Then, I went down to Fletcher's for chai and boiled grains. I didn't feel up to ingesting anything more substantial.

I checked the Posts on my way back to my office. Nothing new on Post One. Post Two had a brief notice of a compromise between the Merchant's Guild and the Fatsos—a Thieves' Market would be opened in Flatlands so householders could redeem any goods lifted over the previous ten days. Typical Lorr deal—the Merchant who sold the stuff got a commission, the Thief who stole it got paid for it, and the householder paid double what the stuff was worth just to get it back.

Post Three had nothing new on the Contramont Miner's Trade Delegation negotiations, and a number of indignant notices about the New Earth Air Service bankruptcy, citing the Delrey Bank as defaulter. I skipped Posts Four and Five and went straight to Post Six, looking for anything on the gruesome discovery behind the Temple of Healing.

Not a thing, not even a complaint about the noise of skimmers or the presence of the City Guard. Nothing about finding the body of a young male, thought to be a student at the Advanced Academy. Nothing, either, about the body of a Licensed Sex Worker found in his own digs. No reason to post anything, I guessed, since the identity of each was known, and the circumstances were being looked into by Admin.

I joined the throng on the Grand Boulevard, passing by the elegant shops and not-so-elegant clet stands on the way to my office. Jake was waiting for me, looking distraught.

"Pola! I sent a message to Fletcher's, but it must have missed you."

"I didn't get any message. What's wrong?"

He led me to the private entrance to my office. I gaped at the sight of the door swinging wide open.

"What the...? Death and Destruction, Jake, what happened here?"

The door had been attacked around the handle with some kind of pry bar. Not that the lock was anything complicated—a well-trained Thief could have opened it with a hair-clip. It was mostly there for show. I didn't expect anyone to target a plain door in an alley lined with them.

"Who did this?"

"I have no idea. Pola, this wasn't supposed to happen. When you took this room, you said you'd have a nice, quiet, private business. I suppose this is what comes of renting to an Independent. No Guild to back your word."

I stepped carefully inside to inspect the mess. Paper all over the floor. My desk drawers open, blank forms scattered across the surface. My file shelf was thrown down, the wall behind it visible but apparently undamaged.

I instinctively reached under the top of the desk to the little compartment that could only be opened by pushing a tiny latch. Whoever had ransacked the place missed that one; my stash of coin was intact.

"When did this happen?" I turned on Jake.

"Some time last night," he stammered. "We closed at the usual hour, no sign of trouble. Holly and I just got here and found…this!" He gestured dramatically at the debris.

"Have you sent for the Guards?"

"What for? They're useless when it comes to the Fatsos."

"This wasn't done by a Sanctioned Thief," I said. "None of Fee M'Farr's people would be so careless as to smash their way in then leave coin behind." I started picking up papers. "This wasn't a robbery, Jake. They were after something they thought I had."

Jake stopped fussing. "In that case, *you* deal with it. I'll send for a carpenter to repair the door, but you will pay for the work. The Construction Guild will charge double for an Independent. And your rent just went up by one silver."

"Fine. Can you spare an apprentice to help me clean up?"

Jake glared at me. "If you insist, I suppose I can spare Zeta. She's clumsy and stupid, and I wouldn't even have taken her into the back room if Holly hadn't insisted on it." He left, muttering to himself, "Why do we bother to pay the Fatsos if they don't deliver? I'm going to complain to the Guild. They're the ones who made the deal with M'Farr. Extra protection against thievery, he said! Ha!"

I picked up more papers. I suppose I was lucky the intruder wasn't a vandal. Nothing was torn, nothing was smudged, no ink spilled or styluses broken out of spite. In fact, it didn't look as if anything had been taken at all.

My small stash of coin was intact. My bludgeon was in its usual position, hanging on the hook on the door. It didn't make sense. Someone had searched my office for something, hadn't found it, and just left. Someone thought I had something they wanted, here, in my office, not in my digs. The only thing I could think of was Zac Garber's journal.

I ignored the pounding in my head and thought it through. Someone badly wanted the journal. They arranged for Zac to go to a party, where Emil was supposed to seduce him and take the thing. Then Emil was supposed to hand the book over to Brutus, who was supposed to take it to the Guard House, where it was supposed to be picked up…by whom? Probably another minion of whoever was behind the robbery in the first place. A lot of supposed-tos that didn't happen because…

Because someone else came along and killed Emil. Was it for the book, or for some other reason? It didn't make sense!

Jakki got the book, and gave it to me. And whoever trashed my office must have thought I still had it, because they'd followed Jakki here and hadn't stuck around long enough to realize I'd passed it on to someone else.

A large female poked her head in the door.

"Jake sent me. I'm Zeta?" She edged into the office, taking care not to step on any of the papers. She was fairhaired and fairskinned, on the hefty side, dressed in the pink smock and trou Jake and Holly provided for their helpers. She looked at the stuff on the floor. "He said you'd pay me extra to help out?"

She had the Flatlands habit of ending each statement with a rising tone, making it sound like a question.

I waved at the paper. "Pick it up, put it into piles."

"Sort it out? I'm good at that, I did it when I was working at the Clothier's Guild offices."

An office drone, seconded to a boutique? Sounded like some kind of Guild intrigue, but none of my affair.

I fished the stash of coin out of its hiding-place and laid some out on the desk.

"If a carpenter comes from the Construction Guild, pay him what he asks, no question. I'll be back some time this afternoon. And thanks for coming."

"No problem," she said. "It's better than handing pins to the seamers."

With that settled, I headed for my next stop. I still had my assignment from the Brain, but first I wanted to find out more about exactly how Joyboy Emil and Boffin Zac had met their ends...and whether the two were linked.

v

The Dark Ones' compound stands at the northern edge of the city, far away from dwellings and shops, behind the Admin bunkers. The carrier only went to the end of the Grand Boulevard. I didn't see any pedi-shaws there waiting for custom, so I gritted my teeth and hiked the rest of the way.

Before I could get to see Dark One Kelvin, I had to go through the usual guff, paying the usual coin to get to the place where the deceased were examined.

Dark One Kelvin was waiting for me, long and lean, hair flying around his head, long robe clinging to his scrawny legs.

"I thought you'd turn up," he said with a smirk. "Your curiosity is commendable. Also inconvenient."

"I have some questions about two of your more recent cases," I told him.

"If you mean the unfortunate sex worker in Fishmarket and the even more unfortunate student boffin in Industrial, so have I," he said. "In fact, I am quite concerned. I have given my report to the appropriate authorities, and it has been ignored. Ignored!"

"You have some doubts?"

"I have no doubts at all." Kelvin snorted. "The Licensed Sex Worker Emil was throttled by a waxed cord. Small specks of the coating were left in the wound. And it is my contention that the Contramont student Zac Garber was throttled by a similar weapon, very likely the *same* one."

"How can you tell?"

This was intriguing. I know the Dark Ones have all kinds of tech from the First and Second ships, preserved over generations, but there's always a question about how much of it still works.

"It is difficult, but not impossible,' Kelvin admitted. "In this case, however, there is concrete proof. The fibers of the cord remained in the wounds of both victims. I have examined them under a magnifying lens. If asked by a magistrate, I would testify that the two were strangled by the same weapon, in the hands of the same person."

"In other words, we've got one killer, not two."

"Precisely. It is my expert opinion that whatever else happened to the unfortunate Contramonter, he was gone before he was attacked by the vampire vine."

"When would you say that was?" Timing was everything. If I could prove Zac was done while Brutus was in plain sight in the carrier, he'd be cleared.

"Before midnight two days ago. The tide was high, but had not reached the cliff face, where the vines are rooted."

"Can you send a signed deposition to Administration Detention with that information?"

"I already have," Kelvin groused. "Yet I have not received a reply. Ignored!"

"I'll see what I can do to speed things along," I said.

He started for the door, then turned. "Have you given any consideration to my proposition?"

"Which one?" I hedged.

"That we mingle our genes, to produce offspring?"

I hesitated. "I haven't given it much thought."

"It is incumbent on every person on New Earth to produce at least one child," he reminded me. "To increase the human population and expand the gene pool." He sounded as if he were reciting from *The Records of Lorr*, the history manual every pubescent receives when they enter Secondary Academy.

"I am aware of that." I wasn't about to tell this supercilious noodle that I'd already fulfilled that obligation, many years ago, and not voluntarily. None of his business, nothing I'm proud of, and something I prefer not to dwell on. Somewhere on New Earth there's a young person with honey-gold skin and green eyes like mine. Not a common combination. I hope they're happy.

"If you change your mind...?" He shuffled his feet, embarrassed.

"I'll let you know. It's nice to be asked, even if the answer's no. I'll give the characters in Admin a jolt. There's a male in a cell who doesn't deserve to be, and there's someone else out there who does."

And with that, I left the place. I had more information than I had before, but not enough to make a definite accusation. For that, I'd have to go to a place where questions get answered.

vi

The Advanced Academy of Lorr is one of the main cultural centers of New Earth. To hear the boffins tell it, it's the sole reason for Lorr's existence. Never mind Admin's insistence that the city's name is actually an acronym that stands for Landing Operations, Rest and Recreation, or the Guilds' claim that the city was built on trading networks and industry.

Oh, no, say the boffins and brains, the Founders came here in search of knowledge, and the only true source of it on New Earth is at the Advanced Academy of Lorr. The ones in Pangkot and Port Chicago are mere adjuncts to the central source of information—the Big Black Box that came on the First Ship, containing the entire history and culture records of Old Earth.

Over the generations, the Academy has grown from a few small prefabs surrounding the Big Black Box to a sprawling complex of assorted edifices, mostly built of local stone and brick and separated by swaths of greenery. Student quarters range from barebones hostels to elaborate lodges. The students themselves come from all the settlements of New Earth, assuming they can pass the examinations.

Most of the Lorran students are from Upper Tier Guild families or have ties to Admin, boffins, or Dark Ones. A really clever and determined mech or tech occasionally makes it over the hurdles the Advanced Academy puts in their path to keep out "the wrong kind". When they do, it makes something of a splash on Post Six. So much for making New Earth a classless society.

I approached the complex with mixed feelings. I'd been a student, many years ago—one of the Admin debs right after the shake-up of the Merchant's War. Admin was not in good favor, the Guilds were showing their muscle. I got targeted negatively for a lot of reasons, none of which had much to do with me as a person. It took me a while to understand I was a pawn in a board game I didn't even know was being played. After I did, I vowed I'd never let anyone else be caught the same way.

Now I began to suspect young Zac *had* been played the same way, and for all I knew, by the same people. I just didn't know why.

I hopped off the carrier and ambled along Academy Way, matching my pace to the passersby. Most of them were teens or post-teens, varied in gender and skin tone. I spotted the Admin lads in their multicolored kilts, all fashionable and loud, and a squad of jockos from South Coast in cotton shirts and trou, skins dark and toughened by the tropic sun. A squad of tall fairskin females, chattering in Norland dialect, brushed past me, acting as if they were on their way to something important.

Who was missing? Pangkoti. They have their own Academy, of course, run by their assorted religious sects for their own Upper Tier. The refugees who crowd Fishmarket are only welcome at the Advanced Academy as servers. All the Pangkoti boffins are kept under the thumb of the Autocrat, who doesn't allow them to leave the settlement.

A few older folk made their way past the students, males and females in standard Lorr garb, mostly cloth jacket and trou, although one male rebel sported a lizardleather jacket. Probably a teacher of literature, trying to outdo his students in fashionable attire, albeit a few years out of date.

I checked the houses opposite the Academy buildings. I wasn't sure if the Strangers Hostel was on Academy Way or in one of the alleys leading out of it, winding their way to Garden Sector. In this newest expansion of Lorr, senior boffins and academics resided next to lower-tier Admin personnel. I also noted the houses sponsored by the various Guilds for the offspring of the Guildmasters' families and friends. If an ambitious tech wanted to rise, that's where they could find lodgings, mentors, and eventual advancement to Guildmaster status.

The largest and grandest of these had no nameplate. It didn't need one. It was Admin, and everyone knew it. I skirted it carefully. No one I knew would be there now, but I still shuddered as I passed it.

At last, I located the hostel designated for non-Lorran students—a large house built of old prefab walls and cinderblocks five streets away from the carrier station. A placard on the front read ***STRANGERS HOSTEL RING FOR ENTRANCE*** in Lorran lettering.

I turned my jacket to reveal the patterned lining, wound my scarf around my head, and pulled the appropriate handle. Somewhere within, a bell rang. After a minute's wait, a young male opened the door.

"Yes?"

"Is dis de Strangers Hostel?" I asked in my best (or worst) Norland accent. "I vish to speak to de one managing."

"Come on in," he said. "I'll get Papa Ruven."

I stepped into a large open space furnished for comfort and convenience, not fashion. Plenty of tables, chairs, couches, different sizes and colors and upholstery. At a large round table, a good cross-section of New Earth's human inhabitants chattered madly in various exotic intonations of Lorran standard. I tried to distinguish who was saying what, but even with Ficus's enhancements, it wasn't easy.

I assessed the group. Three large fairskin females—Norlanders by their speech—in heavy wool sweaters and trou. Three large darkskin males, one darkskin female, all South Coasters, in long striped cotton shirts and baggy trou, heads wrapped in colorful print cloths.

The table was spread with representations of odd-looking creatures and odder-looking sea craft.

"The Krakens' existence is proven!"

"That is debatable. There is no concrete evidence, only anecdotal."

"The reports indicate sentience, maybe even intelligence."

"Not possible. The sailors are being misled by their own desire for validation of mythology."

"But it's clear something got them back to their ship." One of the Norland females sounded quite certain. "We have the reports firsthand. Three sailors brought back from the depths after a storm. They reported being carried by the large beings…"

"But…intelligent octopi? Nonsense! They don't have brains!"

"Maybe they do, but not the kind we have."

"A squid that thinks?" One South Coaster male snorted in disbelief.

"The report comes from three sources, all verified."

"I still say it's nonsense, made-up legends and wishful thinking. The sailors must have swum up from the depths and got tangled in water-weeds. They couldn't have been carried…"

The discussion raged on. I didn't think the story was very likely, either, but New Earth had only been settled by humans for a mere twenty generations, and we hadn't gone much farther than the eastern section of the North Continent. A few intrepid explorers had made it to the face of the glaciers that cut off the two parts of the North Continent from each other. My father's final sailing expedition across the Middle Sea had vanished, never to be seen or heard from again. No one knows what's really under that water.

Of course, there's always speculation. A few attempts had been made to search under the ocean. According to records in the Big Black Box, there had been considerable undersea exploration on Old Earth. Some scribe had even written a tale about it that got reprinted in the adventure mags, and there were plenty of sailors' stories about the ferocious beasts lurking to snatch the unwary right off the deck of a ship. So far, no concrete proof, just stories for students to argue about.

A second group caught my attention, several youngsters huddled together near the fireplace.

"Do you believe it? They're keeping Zac at the Dark One's compound!" That from one of a pair of Norland females sitting on the slouchy couches.

"These people are barbaric," protested the other. "They won't even let his own people know whether he went over the rail voluntarily or not."

"He didn't leave this realm voluntarily," the first female asserted. "I have it from Tessa, who saw him at the beach when she was gathering samples. He was thrown into vampire vines and left to be ingested."

That got everyone's attention, including mine.

"That's awful!" moaned Norlander female Number Two. "He was so happy…"

'No, he wasn't," Number One contradicted her. "He was worried about something. He was writing about it when I saw him last."

"When was that?" I stepped away from my corner. All eyes were on me.

"Who are you? How did you get in?" A Lorran male, clearly the one in charge of the house, had just barged into the room.

I decided on honesty. "I'm Independent Eye Pola Drach. Are you the caretaker here?"

"Drach!" Norlander Number One interrupted us. "Related to Drogo Drach?"

"My father," I said, trying to look modest. Drogo Drach is a name to be reckoned with in Norland.

She looked me over. "You are the one he fathered by the Lorr female?"

I couldn't deny it

"I am Britta Drach, also of Drach blood. We are Kin." She struggled out of the folds of the couch to embrace me. "We must feast on each other. I had not thought to find kinfolk in Lorr. It's been many years since Drogo Drach left us."

I looked her over, trying to estimate her age. At first I tensed, thinking this was the encounter I'd been dreading for so long. Then, I did some arithmetic and decided she was just a little too old. She may well be kin, but she wasn't directly mine.

"That's something we can discuss later. Right now, I'm more interested in young Zac Garber."

"Why are you asking?" the caretaker demanded. "I am Papa Ruven, Mother's Guild. These young people are under my supervision. I was shocked to hear Zac was..." He hesitated, unwilling to say the evil word.

"He's dead." That was a South Coaster male, typically blunt and brutal.

"He is, and he shouldn't be." I looked around the room and raised my voice to include the group at the table. "I've been hired to find out why. Anything anyone knows will help me do this." I dropped the fake Norlands accent. No point in it, now I was unmasked.

Papa Ruven scowled at me. "I won't have my lodgers disturbed," he warned me.

"I just want to ask some questions. If anyone is unhappy with that..." I let it hang in the air. "Of course, if something important comes up, I'd have to notify the Guards."

"The Guards haven't been here," Britta said. "They didn't even think to send a messenger. We'd never have known about Zac if it hadn't been for Tessa."

The entire gang gathered around the big central table while I took one of the chairs and looked them over.

"Now, who's who?" I asked.

They sorted themselves out.

"This is Katri," Britta introduced her friend. "We are studying the organisms of the ocean, and their relationship to those of land. It is important," she added, lest I think she was not being Norland-practical. "Management of resources is critical. And this is Tessa. She is one of the new students."

Katri and Tessa nodded.

Studying sea life made sense for Norlanders. The Conservationists ruled in Norland, where the land froze half of the year. Not a lot to exploit, except the ocean, and there were too many legends of Old Earth and its afflictions for anyone to take oceans for granted, even on New Earth.

"And you?" I turned to the South Coast males.

"Nebo Falar," the biggest and darkest of the lot introduced himself. "There are others, but I am the leader, I speak for all."

"If you say so, but if one of you other lot knows something, now's the time to speak up."

Nebo glared at the others, then muttered something about uppity females. The female South Coaster grimaced; no doubt she'd heard it before, and didn't like it.

"What do you want to know?" Britta spoke up.

"To begin with, when did any of you see Zac last? And was he with anyone when you saw him?"

Britta said, "I saw him when he left to go with some of the males from the Admin Hostel."

"When was this?"

"It must have been…two days ago?" She thought again, then nodded. "Yes, just after I had made my presentation in Literature of the Exploration. I thought it odd that Zac would be in such company. The Admin lads do not usually consort with us. We are too provincial for them." She snorted her disdain.

"Unless they have heard too many tales of Norland females, and want to try their hand at them," Katri added, with another sniff.

"Have any of *you* been approached by Admin lads?" I looked at the South Coast contingent.

"Not we. Too crude, too coarse for those exquisites." Nebo echoed the Norlanders' sentiments.

Clearly, no love lost between the two hostels. Definitely hostile.

"I heard Zac was invited to some party three days ago. Can any of you tell me about that?"

More chatter.

"He didn't want to go," Britta said, finally. "He told me about it. He was not used to female companionship, but he and I were friends, as much as he would let a female be his friend. Contramont is very strict about separation of genders. Males and females are brought up separately, and rarely meet except for religious ceremonies, until they are united for reproductive purposes.

"Zac was uncomfortable in the presence of females, but he and I were in the same class, and we worked together on certain projects. He was fascinated with the origins of plant life on New Earth, and its implications in fossil remains."

I must have looked confused. She elucidated.

"Coal. He was sure he could find more deposits, easier to remove from the ground. And he was convinced that the coal deposits on New Earth were composed of different compounds than those of Old Earth, and that they would therefore have different chemical uses. He had gone as far as using the Academy equipment to isolate some of those new compounds."

I thought of the diagrams in the journal. Some kind of coal-mining machine? A new refinery technique? Whatever it was, it might have commercial possibilities...or it might be just some student's air-dream.

"He wrote it all down in that journal of his," Britta went on. "He was always writing in his journal."

"Was there anything else on his mind? Was he unhappy about his classes?" I turned to the rest of the students. "Was he friendly with any of your lot? Besides the Admin lads, that is?"

Nebo spoke up. "He was not friendly. It is not that he thought himself better or worse, but he was not one to join us except at meals. He did not play music, or dance, or take part in betting games at social evenings. He was very serious. Very conscious of being the only Contramonter who had made it to the Advanced Academy."

"Not a party animal, then. Not one to go cavorting in Entertainment Row," I mused.

"Entertainment Row?" Nebo laughed scornfully. "He would not even come to the musical and comedy gatherings at the Student's Tavern. Far too frivolous for the likes of him."

"He did go to the wrestling matches," Katri corrected him. "He was on the team. It was one of the few things he ever did that wasn't purely connected with studies."

"Didn't join in kickball or two-wheel racing?" I was starting to get a fuller picture of Zac Garber, young Contramont boffin. Stuffy, serious, and not interested in anything but coal.

Nebo snorted. "They don't do kickball in Contramont. And he never quite got the hang of two-wheels, so he walked or took a carrier. Not that he went anywhere but the Academy."

"He went to the prayer meetings at his sponsor's house in Garden," Britta corrected him. "Zac did that every ten days, without fail. He was very serious about his religious obligations."

"But he went to the party on Entertainment Row," I pointed out.

"Only because he had to," Britta said. "He was disturbed about going. He spoke with me about it, when I taxed him with being inattentive at our discussion.

"He had brought his concerns to his sponsor, but the Elder told him it was for the good of the Contramont Miners, and said that Zac had to be nice to the Admin lads because one of them was very important, related to a person who was involved in the negotiations. It would seem impolite for Zac not to attend, when he had been especially invited."

"Really? Zac was specifically asked to attend that party?"

Britta nodded. "So he told me. He was not happy about it, and said he only went because his Elder insisted on it."

"And he told you all this…when?" I let it hang.

"It was the day before he…he went to the Other Realm. We were working on the project, as I said, and he was distracted. I scolded him, saying we would not come up to Instructor Feldman's expectations if he did not concentrate. He told me then he was worried about attending a gathering with some of the other Contra-monters, not students, but miners, acting as guards at the Contramont lodgings in Garden Sector."

That meant he was targeted, just as I'd thought. Emil was hired to seduce him, to get the journal. Who was the paymaster? That was still for me to find out.

Yet while I could understand why Emil might be eliminated, I couldn't see any advantage in getting rid of Zac.

"Did anyone see him after he came back from En-tertainment Row after that party?" I asked, looking around the room.

"I saw him, very late, well after moondown." Papa Ru-ven said. "He was not well. It was clear he had indulged in alcohol and was not used to it. The following day, he went out late in the morning."

"He went back to Entertainment Row to find his journal, didn't find it, and wound up in my office," I recapped. "And that same night he went out again, with the same crowd, only this time he didn't come back. You've given me a lot to think about, young people. Thank you for your time."

"What about Zac?" Britta asked. "What happened to him?"

"He was strangled," I said. "By someone who didn't want him to tell what you just told me."

"Are my lodgers in danger?" Papa Ruven asked about what mattered most to him.

"I don't think so. Not unless one of you saw Zac when he got off the carrier two nights ago."

General consultation, then Britta spoke up.

"No. He went out with the Admin lads, and that was the last any of us saw of him."

"I saw him," the South Coast female piped up, ignoring Nebo's ferocious glare. "I was coming back from… from a meeting," she faltered. "With a friend, from one of the Clothier's Guild houses. As I was coming down the street, I saw two males at the carrier station. I thought one might be Zac.

"I was going to greet him, but the light from the station lantern was flickering, and then I wasn't so sure it was him. The other one was definitely Contramont, with a flat hat. His back was to me, I could not see his face."

"Did either of them see you?"

"I don't think so. The light from the carrier station was dim, and I was some distance away, But I saw Zac, I knew it was him."

"Did one of those Contys kill Zac?" Britta asked.

"I don't know. So far, all I have to go on is rumor, hearsay, nothing I can take to the magistrate or the City Guard." I said. "Thank you all for your time, though." I stood. "If any of you have a problem, come and see me." I told them where to find my office. "I'm in your debt," I added, "and I'll pay it."

I left the Strangers Hostel, sauntering along Academy Way, comparing what the students had told me with what I already knew, heading for the carrier station. Something niggled at the back of my mind, some fact that would tie all these strands together into one nice, tight net to catch a killer.

The afternoon breeze was starting to pick up over the estuary. I got a whiff of mud flats and salt, and something else—expensive musk scent. My follower was back.

I stopped briefly, looked around, and tried to catch a glimpse of him. I saw a flash of someone in a multi-colored kilt, conspicuous in that sea of trou. One of the Admin lads from Smokey Joe's?

Academy Way doesn't have much cover—no shops to duck into, only a few clet-stands in front of Academy buildings. The buildings themselves were guarded by Academy Security; no one was taking any chances of another student's riot like the one that started the Merchant's War. Memories are long in Lorr, and even after thirty years, no one wants another upset like that one.

I quickened my pace, sliding around knots of students and instructors, some standing around arguing, others hustling to classes in the former factory buildings. I noted a squad of Dark Ones in pale-blue tunics and jackets marked with a red-on-white sigil on the sleeve, going against the flow toward the Temple of Healing, narrowly avoiding colliding with the students.

I reached the carrier station. At a kiosk, a wizened male hovered over a selection of snacks in coarse paper wrappers, hot and chilled clet, chai, and mags. I ducked around it and waited for my follower to catch up with me.

When he did, I stepped up to him and tapped him on the shoulder.

"Well, well, well, Gorgeous Gyorgi, as I live and breathe! How's business?"

The youngest of the Delrey clan fairly jumped out of his fancy duds.

"Independent Eye Pola Drach?" It was supposed to be a fierce confrontational demand, but it came out a terrified squeak.

"The same. Where are your friends?" I looked around for his usual entourage.

"Um…they had to go somewhere?" He was totally flummoxed at being caught without the gang or his bodyguards.

"Just as well. I wanted to have a chat with you." I looked around. Just past the kiosk was a small table and two chairs. "Why don't we sit here while we wait for the carrier, and have a cup of something. Clet? Chai? I don't think this place does brew."

He looked around nervously. "I'm not supposed to talk to you."

"Who's to know?" I checked the station. No one was waiting for the next carrier, not at this hour. The students and instructors were at classes, the mechs and techs who served the Academy weren't off shift yet. No pedishaw drivers waiting for fares, not until the carrier was due to arrive.

"Vernor. He knows everything."

"So, he finds out you've had a nice cup of clet with me." I smiled sweetly. "No great deal, just a friendly chat about this and that. What's the worst he can do?"

Gyorgi looked stubborn. "Vernor has ways…"

"I know all about Master Banker Vernor Delrey. Come, sit, and tell me about your life."

He followed me to the kiosk. I waved to the server.

"Clet?" I asked Gyorgi

"Chai…I like chai," he whispered.

"Me, too. Can't stand clet. Two chai," I ordered. I turned back to Gyorgi. "Aren't you a little out of your element, Junior Banker Delrey? I heard you'd already left the Advanced Academy, were doing your turn in Admin before going into the family trade."

"I'm…I was…looking for my friends," he waffled. "Some of them aren't quite finished with classes."

"The ones from Transport and Construction?" I smiled blandly. "I don't think they're anywhere nearby right now. And your other playmates seem to have their own business to attend to. So, why don't you just tell me why you're chasing after me, and why you sent one of your people to break into my office?"

That was a guess, but from the way he flushed, I could see I was right on the money.

"I…I didn't."

"You did, but they didn't find what they were looking for. It's not in my office."

"The journal!" he blurted out. "Emil got it, like he was supposed to, but he gave it to that street lizard instead of doing what he was told to do. He was supposed to hand it over to someone else, but he didn't. Vernor said…" Gyorgi shut his mouth, but he'd said more than enough.

"Master Banker Vernor Delrey," I breathed. "He was the one who organized that little whoop-de-do at Pegeen's."

"He wanted the journal. I'm not sure why. Something to do with the Contramont negotiations, or maybe one of the negotiators. He doesn't tell me everything, just what he thinks I should know."

"So, he set up the party, invited the Contramonters, and asked you to make sure Zac was one of the group."

Gyorgi nodded, red-faced.

The chai arrived in pottery mugs, steaming hot and just a little spicy. I paid the server and, once we were alone again, leaned toward Gyorgi.

"Just how did you come to know Zac? He was a first-term student, not one of the Admin crowd. He lived at the Strangers Hostel. He didn't attend the Academy's socials. He wasn't on the scene at all. I shouldn't think you'd even know he was there."

Gyorgi shifted in his chair. "I saw him at the wrestling matches. He was…beautiful. His body…so well-formed, such musculature!" His eyes glowed at the reminiscence.

It wasn't Zac's face that had enthralled Gyorgi, that was for sure. I hadn't been able to assess Zac's physique through the baggy blue trou, but from the bits I'd seen through the vine, he certainly had the form to attract someone like Gyorgi. Whatever he'd done back home must have involved a lot of heavy lifting and grappling.

"So, you furthered your acquaintance," I prompted him.

Gyorigi grimaced. "I spoke to him after one of his matches. I praised his form, suggesting we meet when he had cleaned himself. He wasn't very forthcoming. He refused my invitations to join me and my friends for dinner at the Admin hostel. It has much better food than the other hostels," he added, to stave off any criticism of his tactics. "I told him he could get a real mammal meat dinner, not fish or fowl."

"Maybe he had other things on his mind than food." More likely, he didn't welcome Gyorgi's advances.

"I know what you're thinking," Gyorgi burst out. "But I could tell he was struggling. He wanted it, I know he did. Vernor said as much."

And Vernor would know, but I didn't say that aloud. Master Banker Vernor Delrey's personal preferences were a source of Post Six speculation, but no one wanted to specify who, where, or when. He'd never made any legal commitment to anyone, male or female.

"So, you invited him to join the Contramont party at Pegeen's," I summed up. "Where Emil lured him into a room for a little fun and games, and in the process, that precious journal got misplaced. How did you know about it?"

"I saw him writing in it," Gyorgi admitted. "I would watch him when he went for morning walks, and at wrestling practice at the gymnasium, and at the baths.

He was so beautiful! What a terrible, terrible thing to have happened, that he should take his own life for nothing!"

"What makes you think he did?"

"Why else go over that railing, fall to the beach?"

"And just how do you know that?"

"A messenger, from Admin. And another from the Temple. Vernor pays to get information."

Of course he does, just like Fee M'Farr and almost everyone else at the tops of the Guild pyramids. Plenty of information going around Lorr, just not always available for the rank-and-file. It helps to have a comm, and the electrics to run it. The rest of us make do with the posts, and the rumor chains.

I took another sip of chai. "It's a pity about Zac, but you can rest easy—he didn't throw himself over the railing. He was gone before he ever hit the vines. Someone took a cord to him. Just like someone did to Emil."

"Emil?" He couldn't hide his distress. "But...I thought that was the Pangkoti Fatso, the one Selva hired from Kunine..."

"The one called Brutus, " I confirmed. "But he's got an alibi, couldn't have been near Emil's lodgings when he was...removed. And how well did you know Emil? He seems to have made some influential friends."

"I...Emil and I..." Gyorgi managed to recover his composure. "We grew up together. He was my dear, dear friend." His eyes filled with tears. "I didn't want to believe it, at that waterfront tavern, when you said he was...gone. Not until I got back to the Delrey Tower. Then Vernor confirmed it—he'd heard from the Guards."

"Your friendship...sometimes physical?"

"Once or twice. Not very often. He was Vernor's servant as well as mine, and after I went to the Advanced Academy, we didn't see each other for a while. But I counted him as someone I could trust, someone I could talk to, not just..." He paused, gulped, and sniffled. "I really, really cared for Emil."

"But not as much as you did Zac," I said softly.

"Well...Emil was hired. Zac...was...would have been... very special." Gyorgi finished his chai and looked around, furtively. "I didn't mean to be so forthcoming. I just hope no one sees us together, talking like this. Vernor would not like it."

For a moment, I could see the frightened little lad under the fancy duds and Admin swagger. Then it was gone, and he was Gorgeous Gyorgi, heir to the Delrey Banking fortune and darling of the Upper Tier younger set once again.

"I'll keep what you told me to myself...for now," I said. "But may I give you some advice? For free," I added. "Stay away from Smokey Joe's. It's not healthy for Admin lads."

The carrier pulled in, and I ran to catch it, leaving Gyorgi alone at the table, staring after me. Just before the carrier pulled away, I saw two males in maroon jackets threading their way through the crowd. Gyorgi was right to be worried. Vernor would not be happy about his little brother talking to an Independent Eye, especially not me.

I didn't know whether Fee M'Farr would be back from his visit to the Detention Center, but his Minion-in-Chief, Ratty, would pass on anything I told him…for a price.

I hopped off the carrier in front of Fatso headquarters, a stark slab of a building in contrast to the elaborate structures across the Central Plaza. This was one Guild that didn't advertise its power or wealth; anyone with business there knew what it was, and anyone else stayed away.

I entered with my usual bravado, headed for Ratty's booth in the center of the main hall. All around me were the usual lowlifes, hardbodies, scrawny specimens, and smug types in cheap knockoffs of expensive jackets and trou.

Ratty hailed me before I got halfway to his desk.

"Oyo, Drach! The Master Assassin wants to see you."

"And I want to see him."

One of the scrawny types led me to a room behind the central hall where I was left to kick my heels until M'Farr hustled in, fuming.

"Where have you been?"

"Eyeing," I said curtly. "And did one of your trainees break into my office? Jake is furious. He's paid the Clothier's Guild fee for protection, and he should get it. That door is going to cost some coin to replace. I thought your people were better trained. Breaking that lock? Stupid!"

M'Farr was taken aback. "Your office? When?"

"Last night. Someone bashed in the door, threw papers all over the place, and left."

He scowled. "Not one of mine. One of the first lessons in Thieves' Training is lockpicking. And we tell them not to leave a mess, since it's a sure giveaway the mark's been had. Amateurs!"

"That's what I thought," I assured him. "And here's another for you. That Contramonter boffin? It's likely he was done by the same one that did for Licensee Emil. That lets out your man Brutus, he's totally clear. I hope you were able to get him out of the detention cells."

"It may take some time—Admin's cracking down on violence." M'Farr glowered at me. "Those Pangkoti recruits aren't helping my people keep the peace."

"I don't think they want to," I said. "They rousted a private party at Pegeen's Pleasure Palace a few nights ago and sent paying customers away, just to make themselves known."

"I'm beginning to think it was a mistake to bring them into the Guild," M'Farr confessed. "They can't keep their whatnots in their trou, they make demands on tavern keepers, and they behave rudely to Licensees. Who do they think they are?"

"Big strong males," I said.

M'Farr didn't seem to hear me. He went on with his rant. "And what's worse? Those street lizards. Taking over Fishmarket, undercutting my Sanctioned Thieves. Bunch of snotty infants, that's what they are!"

"They need a strong leader, someone to keep them in line," I agreed. "But more to the point, Master Assassin, there's someone else playing this game, and it's a deep one. You'll hear soon enough. There's something going on between the Delrey Bank and the Contramont Miners."

M'Farr waved that away. "Nothing to do with the Guild. Master Banker Vernor Delrey and I have a deal. He does his thing, I do mine. We don't step on each other's toes." He shifted uneasily in his seat. Even Master Assassin Fee M'Farr fears Master Banker Vernor Delrey. There are rumors of favors done on each side that wouldn't bear examination from Administration Revenue.

"If that's all…" I got ready to leave.

"That dead boffin. You're sure it's an amateur?"

"It looks that way. Done the same as Licensee Emil, too, so probably the same hand."

"I don't like it." M'Farr's scowl deepened. "Do you know how long it's taken for me to sort things out so Lorr is safe for business? How hard it is to rein in hardbodies with tempers and touchy honor systems? Admin understands, the City Guards leave my people alone, we keep things running. And now…this!" He slammed his hand on the table.

"If it makes you feel better, Independent Eye Julian Hunt is also working on this case," I offered. "There's a good reason she's called the Brain. She'll take care of things, sort it out with Admin, and life can get back to normal."

"Hunt? Who's paying her?"

"The Contramont Miners," I said. "And for what it's worth, Master Assassin, I'm convinced this whole mess revolves around them."

"Then it's none of my concern," M'Farr said, his scowl relaxing. "As long as the Guild isn't involved, and it's not about Lorr, I'm out of it. The Contys can run their own show. We're done here."

And he was out of the room, leaving me with more questions to answer.

Once out of the Fatso Guildhall, I again stood at the carrier station, plotting my next move. Should I go back to my office, go to Arriver's Hill, or just take a break and head for Entertainment Row and my digs?

I decided the office came first. I wanted to see how well my new office drone was working out. Then I'd report to the Brain and get back to Ficus.

A skimmer pulled up in front of me. Before I could react, two large males in standard mech boiler-suits grabbed my arms and shoved me into the back seat. It happened in a flash, before anyone was likely to notice a private skimmer on the street.

One roar of the engine, and we were up and on our way. I clutched the side of the skimmer. Only one family in Lorr painted their vehicles maroon. But what did the Delreys want with me?

ix

Have I mentioned I really hate skimmers? They're noisy, they're flashy, they're very expensive to make and maintain, and only a really experienced aeronaut can be trusted to handle one without crashing into one of the hills that surround Lorr. And despite what the boffins say, I don't really believe a column of air can support all that weight, no matter how fast it goes. I'm always waiting for the electric motor to run out of juice and send the whole shebang downward.

I admit, if someone has to get somewhere in a hurry, like Dark Ones in an emergency, a skimmer is the way to go. And there are parts of Norland that are only reachable by skimmer or airship. But for day-to-day transport, most folks in and around Lorr take the carrier or hire a pedi-shaw, if they don't want to use a two-wheel or their own feet.

In this case, I wasn't given a choice. The two hardbodies outweighed me by far too many kilos. Besides, I wanted to hear what their boss had to say.

Up we went to Delrey Towers, a compound that covers the crest of Striver's Hill. One large building, all stone and glass, featured solar panels winking on the roof and a turbine turning slowly on the tallest point. The first Delrey, who built the original tower, made sure there was a private power source for his stronghold.

Three outbuildings included one utilitarian, two gaudy with decorations. A flat space in front of the tower held more skimmers and pedi-shaws than one person could possibly need, All were painted that penetrating maroon, marked with the three gold circles of the Delrey sigil.

Our skimmer landed next to the others with a bump.

"Nice going, friends," I said.

No answer from the mechs. Either they weren't talking, or they didn't understand Lorran.

"Am I being taken prisoner? Or is this a private chat with the Master Banker?"

The hardbodies ignored my chat. They just hustled me into the central building. White stone on the outside had been carved to resemble fluted columns, glass windows between them.

We entered a vast vestibule, no chair nor a bench to sit on, white flooring, and a staircase leading upwards. Electrics glowed in the walls, making the place look even starker. Nothing broke the sheer whiteness, not a picture, not even a sign or sigil.

One of the mechs grabbed my arm. I shook him off.

"No need for that, friend. Just lead me to the Master Banker. That's why I'm here, isn't it? To have a confab with Master Banker Delrey?"

Again, no answer, just a push toward a door at the very back of the hall. It opened at our approach, showing a small cabinet within. Oho! Delrey rated a lift? The hardbodies hauled me in, and up we went.

If Master Banker Vernor Delrey meant to impress me, he succeeded. Most places in Lorr would have stairs. But if the point of all of this was to wear me down mentally before I even got into his august presence, he had the wrong female. It takes a lot more than a fancy airlift to faze me, even though I could feel my stomach drop as we went higher.

The lift door opened. I was shoved into a vast room with windows overlooking the City of Lorr. The sunlight streamed through, blinding me. I threw up a hand to block the glare. My eyes adjusted to the light so I could see through the windows.

From that height, I got a good look at the city below, sprawling around the bend in the river that led to the ocean on one hand and the mountains on the other. I could appreciate the layout—the Central Plaza, with the Grand Boulevard on one end and Academy Way on the other, alleys running off the main thoroughfares. The Guildhalls on the Central Plaza towered over the lower buildings behind them. I could just make out the fishing fleet returning on the evening tide.

There was the whirr of an electric motor as a blind came down over the window, and I could see the room more clearly. It held one desk and two chairs. Nothing on the walls to break the whiteness.

A male sat behind the desk, silhouetted against the glare. I finally got a good look at the person who'd destroyed my life, not once, but twice.

Master Banker Vernor Delrey. He looked to be at least twice my age, a survivor of the struggles for power in Lorr both before and after the Merchant's War. He wore a jacket-and-trou set that must have cost as much as I earn in a year. Sharp features, blue eyes under white brows, his white hair not colored—he didn't have to look younger than he was.

For all I knew, he might well have been born twenty generations ago, one from the Founder's first generation on New Earth. The First Ship was supposed to have had marvelous rejuvenation procedures, and it's rumored the Dark Ones are still able to perform them…for a price.

He said nothing, just sat waiting for me to make the first move in this game.

I greeted him affably. "Oyo, Master Banker Delrey. How's business?" I would not let this character know my knees were wobbling and my innards were clenching.

He regarded me coldly. "Independent Eye Pola Drach. We do not need to be polite. This is not one of your so-called 'friendly chats'."

I could hear the quote-marks around the words. I responded with one of my blandest smiles.

"You have been interviewing my youngest sibling, Gyorgi." He bit each word out as if it was costing him coin.

"Word gets out fast. I just left him. He was worried you'd find out. I suppose one of your mechs spotted us at the carrier station."

"He should not have spoken to you at all."

"It was his idea to follow me," I pointed out. "He wanted to talk. I just let him do what he wanted. You know all about that, Master Banker Delrey." It was how he operated, opening doors and letting people choose to go in them, or not. Of course, he wasn't above giving someone a push now and then.

"What did he tell you?" He ignored my insinuation.

"Nothing much. I simply asked him about his part in organizing the little gathering at Pegeen's Pleasure Palace for the entertainment of the Contramont Miner's Trade Delegation. It seems to have been quite an event, even made Post Six."

"The party was not supposed to become so...noisy." Vernor admitted that much. "Nor did we expect intruders."

"Not a part of the plan?" I guessed. "But with those Conty boys on the loose, what did you expect? You'd think one of their Elders would be on hand to give them some discipline, but they weren't invited, were they?"

"The Contramont Elders allowed their juniors the opportunity for Rest and Relaxation."

"And that included Boffin Zac? But he wasn't really part of the delegation, was he? It's becoming more and more clear to me the whole affair was set up to get that journal, the one Boffin Zac always kept with him.

"Gyorgi told you about it, and you wanted it. Gyorgi didn't know why, but it must have had some information you couldn't get any other way. Otherwise, why go to so much trouble, spend so much coin?"

Vernor's lips tightened. "You seem to have worked it out, Eye Drach. Well, you are right. I wanted it, and I hired people to get it for me."

"Licensee Emil?" His eyebrows twitched. I was right again. "And then Brutus, to get it from Emil, and take it to the Guardhouse, where one of your mechs could pick it up. Only you never received it. What happened?"

"Someone else interfered." For a split second, a tremor quivered in Delrey's stoic face. Then he was in control again.

"And the book disappeared," I finished the story. "Well, Master Banker, you may set your mind at rest. The book has been retrieved, and it is now in very good hands, quite safe. You really didn't need to send one of your mechs to break into my office to find it."

He didn't bother to deny it. "It wasn't there."

"No, it wasn't. I knew I couldn't read it and passed it on to someone who could. Your informant shouldn't have been in such a hurry to get the word back to you. I passed it on to—"

"Not Administration Security!" Vernor gasped. "If one of their boffins gets it…"

"Oh, no. Not yet. Someone unconnected with Admin or any of the Guilds. In fact, I suspect you should be getting a summons from Independent Eye Julian Hunt at any moment."

"Julian!" It sounded like a curse in his mouth. "You gave it to *her*? Why?"

"It seemed like a good idea. I thought with her Advanced Academy background she could figure out what it said. And I didn't want to end up like Emil or Zac. Someone is really determined to remove anyone who has that journal. At first I thought it might well be you, Master Banker."

"I!" He seemed totally affronted. "I had no reason to…remove…either Emil or the young boffin. Emil was…" He swallowed hard. "I knew Emil…intimately." It must have cost him a great deal to admit that, especially to me.

"I regret your loss," I said automatically.

"Not so much as I. Emil served me well for many years, ever since he came to Lorr with his mother. She was a servant in my house then, and he was only an infant. Under other circumstances, they would have been separated, but I kept him as a companion for Gyorgi. Emil was in my service until he…he decided to leave."

Meaning, he got too old to interest Vernor Delrey physically any more but knew enough so that Delrey was compelled to let him go his own way.

"He seems to have done well," I said, more diplomatically. "He continued as a Licensed Sex Worker, earning a tidy sum, pleasuring older males. Unfortunately, he also seems to have had a loose mouth when it came to his clients. He forgot the first rule of a Licensed Sex Worker is discretion.

"It may come as no surprise to you, Master Banker, that Emil was indiscreet about his connections. I don't think your name was specifically mentioned," I hurried to assure him, "but Emil was not above using what he knew about the Upper Tier for his own advantage."

Vernor sighed. "I warned him about that, but he was becoming quite headstrong. Unfortunate, but that is the way it goes with young males."

"If I may, Master Banker…when was the last time you spoke with Emil?"

Delrey hesitated, then waved his hand. "It is of no consequence. He is gone, and the Pangkoti male who did it is in Detention."

"Not anymore," I said. "He's been released to the custody of the Assassins' Guild. It's been proven that he couldn't have killed Licensee Emil." I wasn't sure if this had been done yet, but it would be.

"Then, who did?" Vernor leaned forward. "And what is your interest in this matter, Eye Drach? Why do you pursue my sibling?"

"Because I've been hired——it doesn't matter by whom —to find out what happened to Emil. It all revolves around that party, and Boffin Zac's journal. Someone's desperate to get it. Any thoughts as to why, Master Banker Delrey?"

His lips tightened. "According to the liaison from Contramont…"

"Elder Mackintosh?"

"Yes, I believe that is his name and title. He told me the young male had found a process for removing more fuel essence from discarded coal—what they call the tailings, from mines that had been abandoned.

"He had shown Elder Mackintosh diagrams of an apparatus for extracting the oil and refining it, sketched in that journal. It would have meant more profit for the Contramont Miners, and therefore, for the Delrey Bank, if we could obtain the sole rights to that process."

"I saw the diagrams and formulas. Couldn't make any sense out of them, but I suppose a boffin might."

Vernor's voice sharpened. "Do you realize what this means? If we could tap another fuel source, we could build larger ships, ships that could combat the crosswinds and tides that keep us limited. We could power larger airships to get over the mountains and across the ocean to the Middle Sea, and explore and settle the rest of the North Continent.

"We could reach the archipelagos! We could expand our settlements, go beyond this one small continent, explore the rest of New Earth, perhaps even get to the petroleum deposits in the Ocean Islands." Vernor rose and started pacing. "For the first time, we could use the information stored in the Ships' Computer. What you call the Big Black Box." The light of the fanatic blazed in his eyes.

"But that's not possible now," I pointed out. "Not without Zac's findings."

"Once we have the information in that journal, someone at the Advanced Academy will surely find a way to use it," Vernor declared. "The process is of inestimable value."

But not to Vernor Delrey, if the Administration took over. The Administration boffins would make the information available to anyone who could figure out what those diagrams and formulas meant. Any project deriving from this discovery would be funded by the Administration, and profits would go into the public coffers, not Delrey Bank.

"Too bad for you, but then, Zac's journal is now in the hands of Independent Eye Hunt, not Admin," I reminded him. "And you still haven't answered my question. What part did you have in placing Licensee Emil at Pegeen's?"

"I did not see or speak with Licensee Emil for at least a week before the event," Delrey said evenly. "Any of my servants will attest to that. On the other hand, my sibling Gyorgi was also…intimate…with him. Perhaps he was instrumental in bringing the two together."

Nothing like keeping things in the family. I got to my feet.

"Are we done here, Master Banker? I've told you what I know and what I surmise. I can't tell you any more than that, and you're not about to tell me any more than you have."

"You may leave. You will, of course, say nothing of this conversation to anyone," he said.

"I'm supposed to report what I find about the Contramont affair to Eye Hunt, who is acting for them," I told him. "But you know Eye Hunt's reputation better than I do. I don't think any of this will wind up on Post Six, but if I am directly asked, in the presence of witnesses in a magistrate's court, I will not lie for you." I looked around for the lift door. "Do I owe you anything, or am I free to go now?"

"You are not a prisoner," he said. "But you would do well to remember that you could be."

"Don't threaten me, Master Banker. It does you no good, and only makes me unhappy. You've already done as much to me as anyone could, short of physical violence."

"That was in the past. A regrettable incident, best forgotten."

"Not forgotten by me," I said. "And not by at least one other. Thank you for your time, Master Banker Delrey."

I turned on my heel and glared at the door. The lift opened. The same two hardbodies waited to take me back to the skimmer.

"Clothier's Alley," I ordered. If I had to endure another ride, at least they could take me where I wanted to go.

They didn't. They dropped me off exactly where they'd found me, in front of the Fatsos' Guildhouse.

And I wondered, What in the name of the Founders was that all about? Who was looking for information from whom? And why go to all that trouble to intimidate me?

I decided to let it go for now. I had other things to worry about.

I stood there for a while as humanity surged around me. The sun had dropped by a few degrees, but there was still plenty of daylight left. I decided to cut across the Central Plaza to Clothier's Alley, picking up a meat-pie from one of the vendors in the plaza on my way.

I actually made it back to my office without being interrupted. A carpenter from the Construction Guild was repairing my door, under the watchful eye of my new office drone, Zeta.

She greeted me happily. "Oyo! Eye Drach1 I've sorted your files, and arranged them neatly."

I've never seen the need for an office drone. I keep my own records, I'm capable of handling my own finances, and if I'm away from the office, Jake or Holly takes my messages. I don't have the coin to pay someone to sit on their hunkers waiting for clients to find their way to my door.

Still, it was nice to step into a space where everything was in its place. Not necessarily the place where I'd have put it, but not all over the floor, either.

"Why did you rearrange the furniture?" I asked.

"I thought the desk looked better in the corner, opposite the cabinet," Zeta explained.

"I liked it where it was, opposite the outside door. And I wanted the cabinet where I could reach it without getting up," I complained.

"The cabinet had been pulled away from the wall anyway. Besides, exercise is good for you."

This was the other reason I don't have an office drone. I don't need anyone telling me what to do. I had more than enough of that growing up in the household of Regina Polaris.

"Were there any messages while I was out?" If I have an office drone, she might as well make herself useful.

"One, from someone called Basher. He wants to see you. And Eye Bonwit sent a messenger to remind you of a meeting at the home of Independent Eye Hunt."

"Did Basher say why he wants to see me?"

"Something about a lad? I can't make out the writing, it's such a scrawl." She handed me a scrap of paper.

Jakki's gone. Meet me at Joe's.

That didn't sound good.

"Good work, Zeta. One more thing. Did you see a mug anywhere in the mess? I'd like some chai to go with my pie."

"I saw the shards of something. I'll get you a mug from the ones Jake and Holly keep for their staff." Off she went, and came back with a steaming cup. She set it before me and stood, expectantly, in front of the desk.

"I like this job," she declared. "It's a lot better than picking up pins and threading needles. My stitches aren't good enough for anything fine, and Holly carps at everything I do. Can't I work for you instead of them?"

"I don't have enough work for a full-time office drone," I hedged. "And I'm Independent, not connected with any of the Guilds. Better stick with Jake and Holly, and I'll call on you when I need you."

She shrugged and sighed. "I really hoped you'd take me on. I like office work, and I hate sewing."

"I'll see what I can do."

I really hoped Holly would be able to use her services in the boutique office. I don't want to be saddled with staff, dependent on me for survival. There aren't enough Independent Eyes in Lorr to make a Guild, and even if the three of us wanted to, what would be the point? Each of us has our own sphere of operations, so we don't need a lot of extras. Basher has Velda, and Julian has Reg, but I do better alone.

I finished my snack and considered my next move.

Eye Hunt was waiting for my report. I'd satisfy her curiosity and make my escape before I had to face another of her meals. I'd go home and tend to Ficus, then deal with Basher. And just maybe I'd get through one evening without having to risk either my tum or my skin.

I checked the door one more time, bolted it from the inside, and used the hidden inner door to get through to Holly's office.

It's a lot nicer than mine, but not much bigger. The sky-blue painted walls display drawings of new designs. One pix showed Holly and Jake getting some kind of award. A screen covered in coarse cloth held swatches of fabric and sketches for new garments pinned to it.

In the middle of all this sat Holly, a lot rounder than me, in one of Jake's neatest jacket-and-trou sets, at a desk that took up the middle of the room. She was surrounded by ledgers and papers with numbers scrawled on them, tapping at a numbering-machine. She looked up at Zeta and me, annoyed at being interrupted.

"I thought I told you—" she started in on Zeta.

"You really need an office drone," I interrupted. "Zeta did a grand job of sorting my papers. Why don't you take a break, and let a professional do what she does better than you?"

Holly grumbled something under her breath about interfering tenants, but shifted some of the papers on her desk to make room for the ledger.

"What I do with my business is of no concern to you, Pola. Zeta's here courtesy of the Clothier's Guild. How I use her is up to me."

"It's a waste of talent, putting her into the sewing-room," I pointed out. "You can use some help here, let you get out into the salesroom."

"I'll think about it. And by the way, I've talked Jake into letting you keep the back room, for now."

"That's very kind of you." It was more than kind. Getting another place would be difficult for me, maybe impossible, given the space considerations in the Business Sector of Lorr. The only other options would be to find something across the river in Flatlands or work out of my digs, neither of which I want to do. Flatland was too far from the action. Entertainment Row was Basher's territory. As for Arriver's Hill, that was way out of my price range.

"But no more rough stuff!" Holly warned me, then turned back to the accounts. "This isn't good. With Selva Delrey out of the picture, and that new fad for kilts, our sales have gone down."

I looked around for someplace to sit that wasn't occupied by paper,

"Too bad Jake won't go along with the current style."

Holly grimaced. "He hates them. The colors clash, the fabric's some kind of heavy cotton, and the kilts aren't becoming any but the most slender and fit of young males."

'But the not-so slender insist on wearing them," Zeta put in. "Has anyone dared to tell them what they look like? Especially from the back?"

"Not if they value their hides," I said with a grin. "Especially not the set hanging around Gorgeous Gyorgi Delrey. He looks fine in a kilt. The rest of them…?" I sniggered at the memory of the Transportation and Construction guild heirs in their fancy togs. "Tell me about Gyorgi. A lot younger than Selva or Devon, isn't he? Just where does he fit into the clan?"

"Oh, yes, Gyorgi. The afterthought." Holly put aside her ledger, always ready to dish dirt on the Upper Tier instead of sticking to business.

"I thought I had that clan pegged. Vernor's Old Gregor's firstborn, or at least, the first one he acknowledged." I eased my rear onto a corner of the desk. "Where did the Delrey money come from, anyway?"

"Trade," Holly said tersely. "As I heard it, the original Delrey was an ambitious tech, created a network of trading posts soon after the Second Ship arrived and set up the settlements that became Pangkot and Norland."

"So, the clan goes back, all the way to the Age of Settlement. That's a long time to stay on top."

"There have been ups and downs," Holly said. "Old Gregor was the most recent up, during the Age of Expansion, before the Merchant's War."

"Way before I was even born," Zeta said.

"A long time ago," Holly agreed. "Old Gregor was like a character out of one of the adventure mags. Took a lot of risks, married a lot of females, had a lot of offspring, in and out of marriage, here, there, and everywhere on New Earth."

"But only four that matter in Lorr," I pointed out. "Vernor, Devon, Selva, and Gyorgi. What happened to the rest?"

Holly shrugged. "Who knows, outside of Admin and the Big Black Box? Old Gregor farmed out the males to outside settlements, got the females attached to various other clans. Vernor he kept at home as an unpaid assistant.

"Devon's and Selva's mother was second-tier Admin, so they were brought up by her family, mostly. And Gyorgi?" She grinned nastily. "He came along just about the time the Merchant's War wound down. His mother was rumored to be some kind of exotic entertainer from the Hinterlands beyond the mountains."

"I think I heard echoes of that when I was at the Advanced Academy. Mostly from Selva, who didn't care much for the baby brother. Some kind of scandal?"

"No one is quite certain who Gyorgi's father really was. He turned up right after Vernor persuaded *his* father to take a rest from business and retire to his mountain lodge.

"Next thing anyone knew, Old Gregor announced he had found True Love and fathered a healthy male child.

"The lad was vouched for by Vernor and brought up in the mountains by Mothers' Guild professionals under Vernor's guidance."

"No chance Vernor could have been involved?" Zeta offered.

Holly and I both snickered.

"Given Vernor's choice of playmates, not deathly likely!" Holly snorted.

I wasn't so sure. "There are ways," I offered. "The Dark Ones and their pet boffins are supposed to be able to do all kinds of things using the Old Earth information and techniques. Upper-Tier stuff, not for the lowers."

"Whatever," Holly got back to what was really bothering her. "Gorgeous Gyorgi is ruining my business. All his followers go to Guernreich for their duds. We're stuck with the Upper Tier Admin, and they are starting to look like dowds next to the younger set."

I slid off the desk. "I saw some young people today. Advanced Academy types from Norland, wearing knitted wool tunics. Nice and warm, patterned stitches. You might consider that as your new line."

Holly stiffened. "Norland wool knits? On my clients? They'd look like hairy mammals!"

"How about boiler suits?" I offered. "Like the ones mechs wear, only in very shiny fabrics?"

"Even worse than kilts!" Holly exclaimed. "No Admin would be caught in sunlight looking like a mech!" She turned back to the ledger, shoving a batch of papers onto the floor.

Zeta picked them up. "Clothier Holly, my specialty at the Guild was filing. I could sort and file these papers for you...?" She ended on a hopeful note.

Holly sighed and moved over. "See what you can make of this mess. I want to have a word with Jake."

I left them to do their paperwork. A pattern was emerging, but I wasn't sure where the design was going.

Maybe it would take a more subtle mind than mine to make sense of it. I headed for Arriver's Hill. Julian Hunt had that kind of mind.

xi

I got to Arriver's Hill with no further interruptions. I could hear the whistle of a large transport making its way down the river, hauling a string of barges behind. Barges loaded with coal, ore, or parts to be assembled in the factories on the other side of Flatlands. Ore from the Mineral Mountains and coal from the Hinterland mines, dug out by mech labor supplied by the Construction Guild, paid for and organized by the Bankers' Guild. Quite an achievement for a place that didn't even have humans in it twenty generations ago.

"Oyo! Pola!" I was jolted out of my musings by Basher Bob, who lumbered up the hill to join me at Juilan Hunt's door.

"Basher! I got your message. What's this about Jakki?"

"I'll tell you about it inside. No point saying things twice."

Reg Bonwit met us at the door and led us directly into Hunt's private room. The Brain was waiting for us, this time decked out in a splashy red-and-white caftan with a red scarf wrapped around her head, set off by a necklace of red coral and white pearls.

The infamous journal lay on the desk in front of her.

She got right down to business. "Report!"

Reg started. "I went to the house leased by Elder Mackintosh in Garden Sector. A very nice residence—two stories, inner plumbing, bath and electrics."

That said a lot. Garden Sector was built up right after the Merchant's War, when a lot of the Merchants who wanted to get out of the center of Lorr didn't want to mix with Flatland mechs and techs. The cottages in Industrial were already claimed by the Academy and the Dark Ones, so Admin gave the Construction Guild the opportunity to expand into what had been waste and farmland.

The result was a sector of snug little houses, each on its own plot, available to anyone who could come up with the coin. In other words, to middle Admin and middle-to-upper Guild, before they tried for Striver's Hill. Getting a house in Garden marks advancement, whether in a Guild or Admin. For an outsider to lease one meant a lot of coin changing hands, and suggested permanent residence. Casual visitors use the lodgings between the Business Sector and Entertainment Row.

Hunt nodded. "Continue."

"Currently in residence, Contramont Elder Mackintosh and his staff, a crew of five males, hefty types, all new to Lorr. They've got their respective Visitors' papers from the Construction Guild."

"Some of them got the neighbors in a snit when they came back from that party at Pegeen's," I put in. "I saw the notice on Post Six."

"I heard them when they passed by Smokey Joe's, on their way through Entertainment Row," Basher added. "Hard to tell how many jammed into two pedi-shaws, howling about a bear going over a mountain. What's a bear?"

"A large Old Earth mammal," Hunt told him. "The song is a nonsense ditty, brought on the Ships. Obviously, the Contramonters are not used to the more intoxicating beverages available in Lorr."

"Young Boffin Zac Garber must have been in that crew," I said. "According to the Mother's Guild caretaker at the Strangers' Hostel, he came in late, drunk, drugged, or both. Not in a condition to do much more than crawl into bed. He must have had one deathly hangover the next morning. He didn't look happy when he came to my office, that's for sure."

"And it was during that so-called party that this journal went missing," Hunt summed up, and turned to Basher. "What have you been able to find out in your research on Entertainment Row? I assume you have been looking into the absurd story told by the Flatlands Force male, Brutus. How much of it is factual?"

Basher rubbed his nose. "I've checked it out. Eye Hunt, this involved some people I do business with, who I don't want to get into trouble with their uppers."

"Rest assured, Eye Basheer, names are not necessary. I only want to ascertain the facts. According to Eye Drach, your client claims he was accosted by an unknown male and given a small sum to obtain this journal from Licensee Emil. He did not do so immediately, but waited until daybreak, at which time he went to Emil's rooms, found him on the floor, and left. Is that the gist of it?"

Basher nodded. "That's what he said. And yeah, I checked it out. I've got a few friends in the Guards. One of them is stationed at the Waterfront Guardhouse. He told me there was someone called at the Guardhouse, claimed to represent a particular Upper Tier Banker, and asked for a small favor. More than that he wouldn't say, but he figured it wouldn't hurt to keep a package for someone with that much clout. So, that part of the story matches what Brutus said."

"A favor?" Hunt echoed. "Can your contact identify this mysterious visitor?"

"Not for the magistrate. But my friend is sure it was a male, and he thinks there was a skimmer waiting for him. He heard the buzz and roar, and there was a stiff wind when he left."

"A skimmer? On the Waterfront? And no one noticed it?" I asked skeptically.

"If anyone did, I didn't find them," Basher said. "According to my friend, the visitor arrived after dark, didn't want to be seen. But there was a skimmer around, the guard was positive."

"And when did this happen?" Hunt asked.

Basher counted on his fingers. "Two…no, three nights ago."

"The night of the party," I said. "The mystery male must have waited by the bridge for Brutus to arrive after he made his deal with the guards. Brutus said he was called out by name."

"Sounds complicated," Reg complained. "Emil gets the book, hands it over to Brutus, Brutus takes it to the Guards, the Guards hand it over to…who?"

"Whoever takes it to the Upper Tier Mystery Male," I said slowly. "But there's something wrong. That's not how Vernor Delrey works. He never does the dirty deed himself, he gets someone else to do it. Puts pressure on them if he can, hires them only if he must. No coin passes, nothing in writing, nothing anyone can point to or hand over to a magistrate. All done by innuendo, suggestion, coded messages."

Hunt nodded in agreement. "I am quite aware of how Master Banker Vernor Delrey operates. I have known him for longer than any of you have been alive." She might have said more, but bit it back.

"So, what happened this time?" Basher asked me. "Why go out and do the deed himself?"

"The information in the journal is so important, he had to make sure he got the right person. He couldn't trust this one to an underling. One of his mechs wouldn't know one Pangkoti hardbody from another, especially in the dark." I allowed myself a small smile. "He knew Brutus, by name and by sight, as one of Selva's crew. Vernor could trust Brutus to do exactly what was asked of him."

"But he didn't," Reg objected.

"Sure he did. Just not right away," I said. "Brutus did what he was told to do, but he took his own sweet time doing it. Showing his independence."

"A mistake on Banker Delrey's part," Hunt agreed and turned back to Basher. "What else did you discover on Entertainment Row?"

Basher looked smug. "You want to know about Emil? Velda asked around the Licensed Houses. Emil came on the scene about two years ago. He didn't do his business connected with any one house, worked here and there, used places like Vassily's Veranda for patrons. Word from Sal is, he was let loose from one of the big houses, maybe Arriver's Hill or Striver's Hill, or even from someone's private lodge."

"Not a street joyboy," I agreed. "More like a special service, available on request for particular clients, especially the ones connected with…" I waited for it.

"Master Banker Vernor Delrey," Basher finished for me. "It took some doing, but Velda found someone who saw a pedi-shaw with the Delrey sigil in front of the Veranda. And who do you think got out?"

"Someone from the Contramont Trade Delegation," I capped his story. "I heard that one, too, but didn't know about the Delrey connection."

Reg smirked. "I wonder what those strictly male-on-female Contramonters would think of one of their own dallying a male Licensee?"

"From what Friend Zac told me, male-on-male is out of the question, sinful, not even to be thought of."

I looked at the book on Hunt's desk. "But he said he'd put his thoughts and feelings into his journal. Is that what all the fuss is about?"

"Perhaps." Hunt tapped the book. "Your client was not a total fool. This journal contains two sorts of information. One is quite straightforward—his research into methods of extracting more chemical essences from waste of played-out mines, and his speculations as to the chemical properties inherent in the strains of coal native to New Earth."

"Master Banker Vernor Delrey made a point of telling me all about that," I said. "He had his mechs grab me off the street, hauled me to his tower, and gave me an earful about how precious this information was, and how beneficial it would be to New Earth Admin in general and Lorr in particular. And he admitted he was...had been...associated with Licensee Emil."

"Unusual for him to be so open about his motivations," Hunt murmured. "And then he just let you go? No threats, no intimidation? Not even a small bribe to keep what you know to yourself?"

"Not even a small hint that I shouldn't talk to you. I would have thought he would make sure I didn't blab his business, but he just shooed me away and had his people deposit me right where they found me, in front of the Assassin's Guildhouse. I was so glad to get out of his tower of power, I didn't question his motives."

Something else occurred to me.

"I'm not sure why this journal was so important. Zac was going to share the information about his coal formula and apparatus with the Academy anyway. He was scheduled to give a talk about it, and lead a seminar. The other students at the Strangers' Hostel knew all about his coal discovery. But what about the rest of the journal, all the stuff about his thoughts and feelings? He was more upset about what someone might read about those than anything else."

"His more personal entries are couched in arcane terms, using an Old Earth alphabet," Hunt said. "Adolescent maunderings, vague hints, nothing concrete, just references to someone younger and someone older, questioning the meaning of desire, and whether it would be right to give in to sinful impulses or resist them."

"Gorgeous Gyorgi was smitten with his looks," I mused aloud. "He as good as admitted he'd made advances on Zac. Zac may not have known what to do about that. What *would* a young male do?" I looked to Reg for guidance.

"He'd ask an older person, a mentor." Reg said slowly. "One of the other Contramonters."

"Britta, the student he was closest to at the Academy, mentioned he was unhappy about what was going down. He'd asked his sponsor, the one who'd recommended him for the Advanced Academy and brought him to Lorr in the first place, about it."

I looked at Hunt for a response. Her eyes were closed. She leaned back in her chair, chewing on her lower lip

"Eye Hunt?" I queried.

"Not now!" Reg herded Basher and me out of the room. "She's thinking, Let her do it. When she's ready to act, she'll summon everyone here for a showdown."

211

"While she's doing it, Basher and I have to find that street lizard Jakki," I said firmly. "He told me he saw a djinn, but who else did he tell? And what happens when it gets back to…whoever the djinn really is?"

Basher frowned. "No reason why it should get out. Who'd believe a street lizard?"

"You never know how far a story will travel," I said. "Basher, we've got to go back to Fishmarket and find Jakki before that 'djinn' does."

xii

Basher and I left Reg to deal with Hunt while we hailed a pedi-shaw and headed toward the river. Most of the traffic was gone, down to a trickle, a few late-working office drones and shopkeepers going home. It was a little early for Entertainment Row; Theater One's farce wouldn't start for at least another hour.

A chilly wind rose off the river, sending casual visitors into the casinos for food, drink, and companionship. It wasn't cold enough to send all the Licensees indoors—that would come later in the year—but for now, custom was slow. They chatted under the lights on the Row, remaining watchful for stray passers-by who might welcome some friendly attention.

I asked the pedi-shaw driver to stop at Foodie Alley. I hadn't had anything solid to eat all day except the meat pie, and I was awash in chai. Looking up at my window, I saw Ficus, and knew I couldn't go ahead until I took care of it.

"Wait a bit." I told the driver.

Before Basher protested, I hopped out and ran up the stairs to my digs. I pulled Ficus away from the window and told it, "I'll give you water and a bit of clet-powder, but I have to go now. I'll be back soon, I promise."

It rustled its few leaves, almost pleading with me.

"I have to go. Really!" I stroked its newest leaflet. 'You're doing well. You are going to be a grand plant, better than you were before."

It tried to give me another shot of pheromones.

"Don't push yourself. I'll be fine" I didn't have time for more. I had work to do, and I couldn't spend any of it right now nursing a plant, even one as dear to me as Ficus.

Basher met me at the bottom of the stairs. He had taken the opportunity to get a skewer of grilled beast for himself, plus an extra for me, together with a small mug of brew.

"Where's the pedi-shaw?

"The driver got another fare. We're better off on foot. Sit down, have a brew, and think things through. We're no good to anyone starving."

He was right, of course. Wherever Jakki was, my hunger wouldn't help find him.

We munched our way through the makeshift meal. Not as fine as what got served at Julian Hunt's table, to be sure, but edible protein, without the attendant spices. As fuel, it did what it was supposed to do.

"So, what's the plan?" Basher asked between bites.

I gave it about a minute's thought . "Where do you think he is?"

"Those street lizards swarm around the Waterfront, looking for a place to get out of the wind," he said. "Any open door, warehouses. Sometimes the clet-stand owners let them roost in their shacks, keeping an eye on things for a bit or two. The Guards don't bother them, so long as the lizards don't make too much noise."

"Jakki's got a following among the street lizards. Let's look for them, and they'll lead us to him."

"Now, that sounds like a plan!"

Basher finished his meat, and we gulped the rest of our brews. I waved to Fletcher to put the meal on my tab, and Basher and I went back to Entertainment Row, refreshed and ready for action.

There wasn't all that much, not on this night. There was the usual audience for Theater One's farce, but the wind held a hint of the rainy season to come, enough to keep most tourists indoors. Moggy was at one stand, Randi and Kira at another, but no listeners gathered in front of any musicians tonight.

I checked the knots of Licensees gathering under the lanterns. They looked up when they saw Basher, then down again when they realized he wasn't alone. None of them paid much attention to the street lizards, and when questioned, none of them admitted to seeing anyone like Jakki.

We passed various taverns and casinos, but the joyboys seemed to have gone indoors for the night. Gorgeous Gyorgi wasn't on the prowl, probably being disciplined by his sibling and confined to the crystal tower on Striver's Hill.

I poked my nose in the door at the Green Dragon. "Anyone seen Jakki?"

No one had.

The Waterfront stretched out ahead of us. Small boats bobbed at the docks, safely tied up. Their crews were in the small taverns nestled between warehouses or in the covered clet-stands. The felines had gone to their lairs, the pteros were back in their roosts somewhere in the spinneys of conifers along the banks of the estuary downstream.

Water lapped at the piers, driven by the currents and wind. Somewhere under the water lurked creatures large and small, with or without scales. Most of the fish in the river were labeled inedible by the Dark Ones, thanks to the factories spewing their waste. There had been rumors of something large and slimy creeping about, but no boffin had ever been able to capture one for study.

"Tide's rising." Basher studied the scudding clouds hiding the stars. "Gonna be a storm tomorrow."

"Winter's on the way," I agreed. "Any sign of Jakki?"

"Not even a whisper. No street lizards in sight. They're all in their burrows, like good little vermin."

He opened his jacket so he could reach the bludgeon at his belt. I did the same.

We trudged along, hands on our bludgeons. Small reptiles scuttled around looking for whatever small edible bits they could find on the riverbank under the piers, or in the spaces between clet-stands..

I saw a glimmer ahead. Electrics lit the Fishmarket Bridge, one of the two river crossings between Lorr and Flatlands.

"There's something going on under the bridge." I caught a glimpse of someone creeping in the shadows behind the tollbooth, too large to be a reptile, too quick to be an adult male.

I moved closer, catching the sound of shrill voices from the riverbank below.

"I'll check it out," I decided.

"Pola, you don't know what's down there."

"Those voices aren't adults', they're too high. I think we've found where the street lizards go at night. They gather under the bridges, for warmth and companionship. If Jakki's's not there, they'll know where he is."

"Lizards can bite just as hard as any other reptile," Basher reminded me. "I'll go first."

"No, you're too big to sneak up on them. Go find your hardbody pals in Fishmarket. Bring them here to the bridge. I'll see if I can talk these youngsters into helping me find Jakki. If they do, fine. If they try to scatter, you and your pals can grab them. Go!"

I didn't wait for his answer. I was certain I knew what I'd find under that bridge.

And once again, I was wrong.

xiii

I followed the sound, inching down a slippery ramp to the bank of the river below the pier . There, I found a small cave, carved under the bridge by the water over the years. I saw the flicker of flames—a fire lit in a small pit, carefully banked to contain its heat. The flames threw shadows across the roof of the cave; I could just make out several small figures huddled together. I couldn't tell males from females in the dimness, couldn't count exactly how many there were.

Jakki stood apart from the group, his hands stretched out toward the flames, clearly their leader.

They stared hungrily at skewers of who-knew-what toasting over the fire. They had been scavenging, grabbing what they could, to share. I couldn't help but feel sorry for them.

No one is supposed to go hungry in Lorr. The Dark Ones have set up feeding stations, and the two Pangkoti temples have their soup kitchens; but no one was looking out for these youngsters. Too old for Mother's Guild creches, too young to be employed, turned out on the loose, they begged, stole, and scavenged what they could.

I stepped into a puddle. The splash drew Jakki's attention.

He whispered to the others, "There's someone there!"

I stepped into the light. "It's me. Pola Drach. You hired me to find out who hurt Emil, Jakki, but you didn't stay around to see if I finished the job. That's not good business, Jakki. You hire someone, you have to trust them to do what you paid them to do."

"You didn't do what I told you to do. You went to the big house on Arriver's Hill," Jakki said bitterly. "My friends saw you. You gave away the book. Emil trusted me with it, and you gave it away. You betrayed me."

"I gave it to someone who knows how to read it," I corrected him. "That's the smart thing to do. If you can't do something yourself, find someone who can. That's why you came to me in the first place, isn't it?"

Jakki ducked his head, the Pangkoti silent *yes*.

"And I think I know who hurt Emil and why," I went on. "But you ran away before I could ask you any more questions, and you didn't stay with Licensee Velda long enough to be safe."

"I'm safe here." He looked around the cave. "These are my people. Soon I will have more."

There was an odd note of triumph in his voice, which had lowered from his previous pitch. He still had the Pangkoti singsong rhythm and cadence, but not the adolescent squeak.

I stepped closer to the fire. I realized there was a bit of fuzz on Jakki's cheeks. He was older than he looked.

"And then what?" I asked. "Challenge Fee M'Farr, take over the Fatsos?"

"Why not? He is old, fat, and smug. I am young and strong."

"He's got powerful friends."

"As do I. But they don't know it yet."

"Of course not," I said. *Stall for time*, I thought. *Keep him talking until Basher gets here with his hardbodies.* "You and Emil were working together, for the good of your friends. Or maybe for the Autocrat of Pangkot?" That was a wild guess. And once again, I was wrong.

"The Autocrat is a swine. He cares nothing for his people. We will rise up against him, you will see."

"You and Emil, working together?" I thought out loud. "He got the coin from his patrons, turned it over to you, and you used it to fund your cause? Through the Pangkoti temples?"

"Emil was useful, but he was reckless," Jackki said. "And he was not completely with us. He tried to play both sides, getting information from one of his patrons to sell to another. This is not the way of the Nameless One! He paid the price for his deceit."

"The one who killed him, the big male, the one you called the djinn. You think it was one of those patrons, the ones he blackmailed, that had him killed?"

"Who else? I did not want Emil gone. He was no use to me dead." Jakki sneered. "Alive, he could find out things, tell us who was going away for a while, whose house was unguarded, where we could find good things to steal and sell. We do not need the Fatsos, we are our own Guild!"

"If you're out to challenge Fee M'Farr, you've got a problem. He's the one who united the Thieves and Assassins into one Guild in the first place. It took a lot of doing, and he's not about to give way easily. You'd do better to negotiate. In fact, I'd be willing to help you do it."

"He is old," Jakki repeated. "He grows soft. He does not like to fight."

"Don't be too sure," I warned him. "Running the Fatsos is harder than it looks, and M'Farr's been on top for a long time. He's got Admin on his side, as long as he keeps things peaceful. He's got the other guilds backing him. He's kept his people in line since the end of the Merchant's War, and he's not about to let go without a fight. Do you really want that?"

"I have help, too. There are many here in Lorr who will follow someone like me, someone who will get them out of the cellars and into the light. I do not charge outrageous fees to allow my friends to do what they must to survive. It is not the way of the Nameless One!"

Founders' Faith, a revolutionary fanatic! All Lorr needs —another philosophy to argue and fight over.

"So says Ishka Kunine?" I put a sneer in my voice, thinking frantically, *Where is Basher?*

I had been so focused on Jakki, I had ignored the others. Now, hands grabbed me from behind. I reached for my bludgeon, but one of them nimbly unhooked it.

"Hit her!"

"Kill her!"

"She betrayed us! She will lead the Guards here!"

Shrill voices cried out in vindictive fear.

"No." Jakki motioned to whoever was behind me. "Tie her up. Take the jacket and shoes. We can sell them, use the coin for food. We will not kill her—it is wrong to kill. We will let the river spirits do with her what they will." He pointed to the cave's exit. "Put her under the bridge. We will let the tide take her away."

Scrawny prepubescents crawled all over me, pinching and punching, stripping off my jacket and shoes. I tried to fight back, but they were like the lizards in the fish market, quick and sly.

My wrists and ankles were bound with river-vines, prickly and tough. Then, they yanked my arms over my head and tied me to a strut under the bridge, just past the waterline with my bare toes in the water. Then, they left me alone, with the tide rising around me, counting on the rush of the waves and the drone of the passing traffic to drown out any cries for help.

xiv

I don't know how long I hung there. I tried to wriggle free, but those vines dug into my wrists—whoever tied them knew exactly what they were doing.

Kicking didn't do much good. I couldn't get any traction. My arms ached, nearly pulled out of the shoulder joints. I could feel the water rising around me, buoying me up at first; but it was only a matter of time before I'd be too tired to fight the current. I'd just hang there, and the water would cover me.

I tried to cut the vines by rubbing them against the girders above me, but they weren't iron—they were ironwood logs, those tough native trees that absorbed metals from the rocks in which they grew. No sharp edges to erode, not even rough edges for friction. Smooth bark, made slippery by algae and other water plants.

I was only wearing myself out, and I soon stopped.

Then I tried inching down until my feet could touch the river-bottom. That got me closer to the riverbank, but provided no traction. The mud between my bare toes squished, and I couldn't manage to stand in it. Instead, I found myself sinking deeper. No help there.

Centimeter by centimeter, the water covered first my feet, then ankles, then knees. The tide was rising faster and faster, driven by the approaching storm. It reached my waist, over my chest, and still no Basher!

What happened next doesn't make much sense, but I swear by all the Founders that it did happen.

I felt something nipping at my feet. At first I thought of the carp, fish from Old Earth that had been let loose when the First Ship got here. They're fierce predators, growing to huge sizes, only kept in check by the even huger reptiles in the oceans. Some had gotten into the rivers, nearly wiping out local species. One of those would make a short meal of a helpless mammal like me.

I waited for the sting of a bite. Instead, I felt a cautious touch from something slithery and smooth around my ankles. Then, a sucking sensation, and a weird loosening of the bonds on my feet.

The touch went up my legs, around my waist, across my front. A long, dark tentacle reached out from the water, wound around my arm to the wrist.

In the light from the bridge, I could just make out a large, bulbous head that bobbed up and stared at me with great, round eyes. Another tentacle picked at the vine on my wrists, loosening it until I could slip my hands out.

And then whatever it was slid away, back into the river, and was gone before I could even thank it.

I remembered the youngsters at the Advanced Academy had been arguing about the idea there might be intelligent life underwater. I'd heard the legends of the Kraken during my stay in Norland, and the stories of sailors who swore they'd been helped after a shipwreck by mysterious underwater beings with many legs and huge heads.

Still, the First Ship surveys hadn't found signs of any civilization on New Earth, and the Founders had decided there wasn't anything more intelligent than an avian on the planet, making it acceptable for settlement by us humans.

I couldn't say whether the lifeform I encountered was intelligent or just curious. Why it decided to help me, I couldn't say, either. But I resolved never to knowingly eat another cephalopod again.

Once freed, I slid down into the river. The cold water shocked me out of my stupor. I couldn't move my arms very much—both hands and feet had gone numb—but I managed to wriggle and splash my way around the bridge to the solid bank. I was shivering with cold, my arms wouldn't work, I could barely croak a plea for help as I heard footsteps over my head.

Strong arms lifted me out of the water. That was the last I knew for quite a while.

THE EYES
HAVE IT

I STRUGGLED FOR CONSCIOUSNESS IN A BED THAT WAS not mine, in a room filled with beeping mechanisms, with a female Med Tech hovering over me. My mouth was dry, my head ached, my shoulders screamed, and my arms sprouted some kind of tubing. I generally felt as if I'd been eaten by a sea reptile and spat out on the shore.

I managed to croak out what should have been "Where am I?" but came out as "Awk!"

The Med Tech announced, "She's awake". She inserted a glass tube into my mouth. "Sip slowly."

I sucked up some kind of watery sweet syrup mixed with sour fruit juice. "How long...?"

"You've been here since yesterday," she said. "You were brought in by skimmer early in the morning. You've been medicated, your wounds have been attended to, and you've had the requisite inoculations against river parasites. You should be quite well in a few days."

"I haven't got a few days," I protested. "There's a gang of street lizards out to wreck Lorr, and there's a killer on the loose..."

"None of which is your concern at the moment." The Med Tech had been replaced by a full-scale Dark Medico, a female of middle years in the usual pale-blue tunic and trou. "I am Dark Medico Macoy. You are in the Temple of Healing. A private room, no less. Your patron insisted on it."

I took another sip of the liquid. A private room at the Temple? That takes not only coin but influence. Regina Polaris flexing some muscle, no doubt, but I wasn't going to turn it down. Having a parent high in the Administration can have its uses, and if the Chief of Security for the whole planet took the time to secure medical treatment for an erring child, who was I to complain?

"Can we allow Independent Eye Drach to have visitors?" the Med Tech wanted to know. "They have been waiting in the visitors' lounge to see if she is still alive."

"Visitors?" My voice was gradually coming back. "Who?" I wasn't expecting Polaris, but you never know. She might have set aside a few moments in her schedule to see what trouble I'd got myself into.

"Two males—they call themselves Independent Eyes. Bonwit and Basheer."

Reg and Basher? Hanging around at the Temple of Healing? Most Lorrans stay far away from the place unless they absolutely need it. I guess we Eyes have to stick together, even if we don't have an official Guild.

The tech added, "They wish to speak to Eye Drach as soon as she is awake."

"I'm awake," I could form words, and my throat was unsticking, but I shifted uneasily. I really needed to use the "place"! "Can I get unhooked from these things?"

"Since you are awake, I suppose you can take nourishment by mouth," Medico Macoy decided. She gave the Med Tech a series of orders that made no sense to me, but the Tech proceeded to remove the various tubes and needles, and covered the resultant minor wounds with gauze.

I struggled to lift myself out of the bed…and realized I was wearing some kind of shirt, open in the back, that reached somewhere around the middle of my thighs. The rest of me was open to view.

"Clothes?" I looked around the room. "Where are my shirt and trou?"

"What you were wearing was sodden," the Med Tech said. "Your friends brought some garments for you." Her voice dripped with disdain.

I had to admit, she was probably right. Velda had likely just grabbed whatever was handy out of my clothes-press, the result being a mismatched blue jacket and gray trou, a yellow shirt, and the usual under-pinnings. The best you could say about the ensemble was, it was clean and not wet.

"I need the…" I let it hang.

"It's here. I'll help."

A private facility? This was luxury on a grand scale. Someone was really spreading the coin, but who? I only hoped I'd manage to repay the debt without going into total bankruptcy.

By the time I'd taken care of personal needs and gotten back into bed, the machinery had been removed from my room. The Med Tech sorted me out, straightened pil-

226

lows, and made sure I was comfortable before admitting my visitors.

Basher stormed in, followed by Reg.

"Pola! I thought you'd wait until I got back."

"What took you so long?" I accused him. "I was hung up under that bridge."

"I had to get to Fishmarket and round up the fellas," Basher explained. "And then when we got there a swarm of street lizards came out from under the bridge, and we had to beat them off. That drew the City Guards, and we had to explain to them, and by that time, the lizards had scattered.

"Then it was dawn, and some fisherman said there was a body coming up from under the bridge, and that it was you." He paused for breath. "So, the Guards called the Dark Ones, since you were still breathing, and they took you to the local Shrine. Next thing I knew, you were being hauled off in a skimmer…"

He glared at Reg, who took up the thread.

"Your name came up on the daily comm transmissions to Admin Security. Eye Hunt sent a private message to Security Chief Polaris, and was told to go ahead and get you treatment. Between the two of them, you were brought to the Temple of Healing, placed in private treatment, and here you are."

"Friends in high places," I murmured. "I wasn't aware Eye Hunt and Security Chief Polaris went back that far."

"Neither was I," Reg admitted. "But there are a lot of things I don't know about Eye Hunt. What's important is, she wants to see you as soon as you're able to move on your own."

I swallowed more of the liquid. Whatever it was, it worked. I was finally able to think clearly, and even articulate what I thought.

"You may have to negotiate for me," I told Reg. "But I'll be out of here before moonrise tonight." I looked at Basher. "Ficus? Has someone taken care of my plant?"

"You nearly drown, your arms get pulled out of their sockets, and all you can think of is that futtering plant?" Basher exploded. "I thought you'd really done for yourself this time. You had water critters crawling all over you, you were nearly gone, and all you care about is that weed?

"Be easy. Velda gave the scrawny thing some water and a spoonful of that clet stuff when she went up to your digs to get your clothes. The river water ruined your outfit. What happened to the jacket? That was good material!"

"It'll probably show up at a booth in the Thieves' Market," I said philosophically. "I'll have to get another one." It wouldn't be easy to replace. It was one of Jake's newest designs, with one of the new metal zip closings so much better than buttons that keep coming loose. "I just hope those lizards got a good price for it.," I added.

I was able to snark. I was on my way to recovery.

Dark Medico Macoy arrived with a squad of Dark Ones and med Techs. They shooed Basher and Reg out and proceeded to give me a thorough going over, checking to see if all my insides were still working and my outsides hadn't suffered more than cuts, bruises, and abrasions.

By the time they were finished, I'd had enough.

"I'm leaving," I announced. "I can walk on my own, I'm in a fit state of mind. I'm grateful for all the fine care you've given me, but I have things to do, and I can't do them in the Temple of Healing."

"Holy Hygeia will not like it," the Med Tech warned me. "It will send evil upon you."

"I'll deal with that when and if it comes," I told her. "Right now, I want some fish soup, roasted root-veg, and a hearty mug of brew. After that, I have to stop a killer from striking again."

Reg and Basher were waiting for me with two pedishaws when I finally got out of the Temple of Healing.

"Basher, you take that one." Reg took over. "Pola, you're with me. Eye Hunt is waiting, and she's set up one of her charades for tonight. It will all be settled then."

ii

I wasn't quite as fit as I'd told the Dark Medicos I was. My arms still hurt, my back was worse, and I was a little wobbly on my feet; but I was able to make it into a pedi-shaw without falling. Reg took my arm and assisted me into the seat. I leaned back, grateful for the opportunity to rest while the driver negotiated the usual traffic on the Grand Boulevard.

Once at the Hunt's house on Arriver's Hill, Reg escorted me to a small room in the rear, where a table had been set up with a set of eating utensils.

"Eye Hunt sent some nourishment for you," Reg explained. "Take it from me, Freddy's soup will restore you to health better than anything they pumped into you at the Temple of Healing. Tuck in, Pola. Eye Hunt has already dined, and will let you know when your presence is needed.

"Meanwhile, you can see and hear everything that goes on if you peek through this opening." He moved a picture of a waterfall aside to reveal a window just about my eye level.

Reg left me to eat my meal. He was right about the soup—it was some kind of fowl, not fish or reptile, with noodles and bits of root-veg to thicken it. There was bread and cheese on a plate next to it, and a mug of really fine brew. When I was finished, I felt better than I had in days. Whatever Cook Freddy had done to it, that soup was definitely the Prime Restorative!

The sound of angry voices in the next room drew me to the peephole. Quite a crowd! I could only guess at the debts that had been called in to get Vernor and Gyorgi Delrey in the same room as the total membership of the Contramont Miners Trade Delegation and Master Assassin Fee M'Farr, with his faithful sidekick Ratty. Captain Sara Atterson and two of her Special Squad appeared to be overseeing the lot of them while escorting Fatso Brutus. They filled the room, large as it was. Atterson had to stand by the door so the bigwigs could occupy the chairs.

I could hear more voices in the hall. Everyone had brought reinforcements. Conty bodyguards, Fatsos, Delrey mechs. I could almost smell the testosterone from my little hidey-hole.

The only ones missing were Basher and Jakki. I assumed they'd be making their appearance shortly. The Brain wasn't about to leave them out of the mix.

Hunt swept into the room, gave me a quick nod, and proceeded through the inner door into the library, taking her place at the desk with Reg right behind her. She greeted the assemblage with aplomb.

"Thank you for coming. I realize all of you are busy people, and I apologize for interrupting your evening activities, but I feel this matter cannot wait any longer. Too many lives have already been lost."

The Contramonters all started yelling. Fee M'Farr growled something under his breath. Vernor Delrey just looked as if he smelled something rotten on the estuary flats at low tide.

Hunt held up a hand. The hubbub quieted.

"I begin by stating this is by no means an official hearing. If, in the course of these proceedings, illicit activity is revealed, Captain Atterson of the City Guard is here to take the appropriate action. What is said and done here may or may not be used later as evidence before a magistrate, but for now, let us assume this is a private meeting."

"You are quibbling, Julian, and you know it," Vernor Delrey protested. "I was not invited here. I was forced. By what right do you summon me to this…" He looked around the room, but failed to find the appropriate word to describe the assorted lower-tier males surrounding him. It struck me that the only females in attendance were Atterson and Hunt. And me, but I wasn't a part of the action. Not yet.

"I am sorry to have to use extreme means, Banker Delrey," Hunt said, "but your presence is necessary to unravel a series of events that have led to the demise of two persons."

"Persons?" Vernor sneered. "What persons?"

"I refer to the Licensee known as Emil, and the student boffin from Contramont, Zacharias Garber."

"Brother Zac's death was accidental," Elder Mackintosh protested. "The Dark Ones pronounced it so. It was recorded by the City Guard."

Atterson spoke up. "Dark One Kelvin's latest report corrects the first finding. It is now certain. Boffin Garber was strangled before he went over the railing."

"Unsanctioned!" Fee M'Farr had to have his say. "Not my doing, nor any of my people!" He glared at the rest of the company.

"An amateur," Hunt agreed. "But one with a knowledge of techniques for killing."

"What has this to do with us?" Elder Mackintosh blustered. "We are not citizens of Lorr. We are free and independent citizens of Contramont. We do not consider ourselves bound by Lorr Regulations."

"Elder Mackintosh, be still," Elder Pinckney admonished him. "As long as we are resident in Lorr, we must abide by their laws." He turned back to Hunt. "You sent a message to our residence that you have solved the problem we set before you. How does the sad fate of young

Garber pertain to the missing funds? Surely, he did not take them."

"He did not," Hunt said. "But he discovered who did, and that led to his demise. He wrote everything into his journal. This journal."

When she pointed to it, all eyes fixed on the leather-bound book on the desk.

"I must digress for a moment," she continued. "This is a somewhat tangled account, with several strands of narrative and mixed motives."

"I do not see what this has to do with me," Vernor Delrey insisted. "I never met this young male, Zacharias Garber. I know nothing about him."

"Oh, but you did," Hunt corrected him. "Your sibling, Gyorgi, was obsessed with him, and you keep a careful eye on Gyorgi's activities and monitor his companions. You knew about this journal, and your liaison with the Contramont Miners' Delegation informed you of the discovery of the chemical properties of the coal found in the Contramont mines.

"And you certainly knew Licensee Emil. You admitted it to my colleague, Independent Eye Drach. I can summon witnesses, if necessary, to attest to just how *well* you knew Licensee Emil."

Vernor's pale face took on a tinge of pink. "Since you have pried into my private life, I cannot deny my… acquaintance with Licensee Emil. He was one of my servants at one time. However, you will also find he left my employ some time ago to pursue a career as a Licensed Sex Worker. What of it?"

"He may have left your household, but he never left your employ. I strongly suspect you used Licensee Emil's services in various schemes. You introduced Emil into social gatherings where he would ingratiate himself with delegations seeking favors from the Delrey Bank. I also suspect this is how he connected with a member of the Contramont Miners Trade delegation. "

"What!" Elder Pinkney was outraged.

"Sad to say, not all Contramonters are as righteous as you, Elder Pinkney," she continued. "Some are more amenable to vice than others, and both young males and their elders can be tempted to enjoy the pleasures of the flesh. Master Banker Delrey provided some."

"An orgy!" Elder Pinkney exploded with wrath. "A vile display of females, fueled with alcohol and narcotics, to lure our young people from the path of righteousness! I told you not to allow them to attend such a function!" He aimed his fury at Mackintosh, who turned pale, then red under such a barrage.

"It was only a party," was the best excuse Mackintosh could come up with. "A friendly gathering, with food and drink, and some companionship."

"And not only female companionship," Hunt went on. "Junior Banker Delrey became infatuated with Zacharias Garber. He thought to seduce him into behavior that went against Contramont customs, using Emil as a conduit."

All eyes were now on Gorgeous Gyorgi, who squirmed in his seat.

"It was all Vernor's idea!" he blurted. "I suppose someone saw me at the wrestling match—he's got spies everywhere—and the next thing I knew, he'd hauled me up to the tower for a little 'chat'." Gyorgi grimaced. "He went on and on about the negotiations with the miners, said how stubborn they were, wouldn't concede an inch, insisted on full rights to all products of the Contramont Mines.

"Vernor had some kind of arrangement with the resident liaison, but there was a whole new delegation, and he wanted something to hold over them."

"I assume the liaison in question was Elder Mackintosh?" Hunt asked.

"He didn't say the name, only that he was more amenable to compromise than these new people. That was when Vernor brought up the possibility of getting some dirt on them, something that would make them more willing to give the Delrey Bank more influence on the Contramont Mines."

"The negotiations? Hah! There were no negotiations, only demands!" Elder Pinkney exclaimed. "The Delrey Bank would have taken control of the total output of the Contramont mines, taking sixty percent of the gross profit. They would dictate the terms under which we would ship our ore, to which settlement, to which refinery. We would be perpetually in debt to that bank, with no recourse to any other funding."

"And any results from Boffin Garber's discoveries would be under the control of the Delrey Bank, to be disbursed or not, as they saw fit," Elder Kennington added.

"It was simply unacceptable. I do not know why you even considered such a contract, Elder Mackintosh."

Hunt tried to take control of the discussion again. "The particulars of the contract are immaterial, as is the import of young Garber's findings, or the efficacy of the apparatus he designed to extract the essence from coal. What is important to this investigation is that Banker Vernor Delrey learned about the journal, and Licensee Emil was employed, or persuaded, either by Banker Vernor Delrey or Banker Gyorgi Delrey, to seduce Zacharias at Pegeen's Pleasure Palace, and obtain said journal.

"On that same evening, someone accosted the former mercenary, now Flatland Force Brutus, on his way back from his rounds, gave him coin, and ordered him to obtain the book from Emil. Brutus was then to hand the book to one of the City Guards stationed near the Fishmarket Bridge, who would turn it over to someone else, who presumably, would get it to Banker Delrey."

"Sounds complicated." Atterson visibly struggled to follow the thread. "And it's all speculation."

"But you like complications, Vernor." Hunt used his first name like a curse. "It's just the sort of thing you do, keeping yourself well away from the unpleasantness of action.

"And one part of the chain required your direct participation. No one else could identify Brutus by sight, and you couldn't trust anyone else to do your bidding." Hunt turned to where Brutus stood behind Fee M'-Farr. "Force Brutus, have you seen or heard anyone here who you recognize?"

"Him." He pointed to Vernor. "I never saw his face, but that's the voice I heard. He gave me a purse, told me to take the book from Emil and bring it to the Guard House. And I would have, but Emil was done when I got there. And that's the truth, by the Sacred Word of Mata Diva." Brutus folded his arms and stared defiantly at Vernor Delrey.

"And that, Master Banker Vernor Delrey, puts you personally at the scene of the action," Hunt said. "Unfortunately, none of what you have done constitutes a crime under the Regulations of Lorr. Your behavior is reprehensible—unethical, even—but not illegal. Your scheme failed, and I recommend the Contramont Miners to take their business elsewhere."

"And what about our missing funds?" Elder Pinkney objected. "Where is our money?"

This was my cue to take action. I stepped through the door, made my way through the crowd to Hunt's desk, and announced, "I can tell you all about that, friends. And it all begins and ends with Emil."

iii

All eyes were now on me. I wasn't looking my best, in that tatty jacket and trou, with half my hair in a knot at the back of my neck and the rest falling into my eyes in front. I waited until the inevitable hubbub died down.

"Independent Eye Pola Drach," the Brain introduced me. "You may now explain how you came to be involved in this sad affair."

"Boffin Zac came to me four days ago," I stated. "His story was, when he awoke the day after the party at Pegeen's Pleasure Palace, he noticed his precious journal was missing. His first thought was he'd misplaced it at Pegeen's, so he went to find it. When he couldn't, one of the Licensees pointed him at me."

"And you took on the task of finding the journal and returning it to its owner," Hunt summed it up.

"I did. And I traced it to Emil. But when I got to Emil's rooms, he was already..." I hesitated, not wanting to say the evil word. "Captain Atterson can attest to that."

Atterson nodded. "I was there. So was Drach."

"But not the journal," I said. "I reasoned that Emil was no fool—he'd hidden it somewhere. Before I could go after it, along came his servant Jakki claiming he'd seen the one who'd killed Emil. Everything pointed to Friend Brutus, so I went after him—"

"I didn't do it! I didn't do the joyboy, and I didn't do that Conty, either," Brutus burst out. "I left him at the carrier station, and went back to Smokey Joe's. Ask Basher, he'll tell you."

"Eye Basheer will join us presently," Hunt said. "Continue."

Brutus went on. "I went back, like I said. By that time, they'd settled things with those two singers. We sang some of our songs, and they sang some more, and it was nearly morning when me and my pals got back to our own house. I went to sleep and didn't get up until the priests came to chase the spirits away from the house where Emil was killed."

"This is very confusing," Elder Pinkney groused. "What has this person to do with our dear Brother Zacharias?"

"Here is where the two parts of this yarn get tangled," I explained. "When I went after Friend Brutus at Smokey Joe's, after I was done with Jakki, I also saw Friend Zac, tagging along with Junior Banker Delrey and his cronies. I felt the Delrey connection was a bad influence on an innocent lad from Contramont, so I extracted him from their company and sent him on his way back to his own hostel." I stopped for a breath. "It was a mistake. I admit it. I had no idea I was sending him from a bad place to a worse one."

Hunt said, "It would have made no difference, Eye Drach. Boffin Garber was doomed as soon as he spoke to the one person he trusted. The one who had brought him to Lorr, who wanted to use his discovery for his own purposes."

The two of us turned to the Contramont delegation.

"Elder Mackintosh," I said, "I don't know what Friend Zac saw or heard, but he was puzzled. He came to you with questions."

"You cannot know what was in that poor lad's mind," Mackintosh scoffed.

Hunt tapped the book on her desk. "Oh, but we can. He wrote his misgivings in his journal. He wrote in a private code, using obscure terms in an ancient alphabet, but the meaning was clear.

"He observed you in conversation with a dubious person in Delrey livery, who handed you something, possibly a purse, possibly a draft on the Delrey Bank.

"At the same time, Junior Banker Delrey was being unusually attentive, hovering about him, inviting him to join his coterie. Both of these things made the young man apprehensive. He took his difficulties to his mentor—you, Elder Mackintosh. He did not know how to deal with Junior Banker Delrey's interest.

"In his journal, he suggests you were dismissive of such matters. He also wondered if you were secretly in the pay of the Delrey Bank, trying to shift the negotiations in their favor. Both these things were causing him great anxiety."

Elder Pinkney's face grew grimmer with each word. "Bribery! Our own representative, conspiring to rob us!"

"I don't think Friend Zac's ethical dilemma mattered much to Elder Mackintosh." I turned my gaze on the agitated Contramonter. "*He* was more concerned about Emil, and *his* demands."

"Emil? The Licensee? And Elder Mackintosh?" Elder Pinkney gasped. "Sinful behavior!"

"All too true," I assured him. "I have at least one witness ready to swear she saw Emil and a Contramonter entering a certain establishment used for private meetings."

Hunt got in another dig. "I believe, if you double-check the financial records of the Conrtramont Miners' account at the Delrey Bank, you will find the missing sums were removed by Elder Mackintosh for 'personal expenses'. Those were not the day-to-day expenses of running the household, but payments to Emil."

There was a collective gasp from the Contramont Elders.

"Emil had some very expensive togs, and what didn't go on his back went to the two Pangkoti temples," I added. "The priests said he was generous, which is all very well—a lot of poor folks get fed by the soup kitchens. But do you really want to fund pagan temples, Elders?"

While I paused for breath, Atterson moved closer to Elder Mackintosh, and the rest of the Contramont Miners tried to shift away from him.

I went on. "Junior Banker Delrey says it was Master Banker's Delrey's idea to stage the party at Pegeen's and lure young Zac to it. Master Banker Delrey wanted the journal for its information, Junior Banker Delrey wanted Zac to taste forbidden pleasures, and Elder Mackintosh wanted…what, Elder Mackintosh? How did you feel when you found out exactly who Banker Delrey had hired to seduce young Garber?"

Elder Mackintosh turned on Vernor Delrey with loathing. "Emil told me himself. I had a…a meeting with him…"

"At Vasily's Veranda," I said. "You were careless, you allowed yourself to be seen."

"I had met with Banker Delrey earlier. He told me what to do, that he would extend me more credit if I got young Zacharias to go to the gathering at Pegeen's. Then he dug in the knife, saying he'd got one of his best servants to abstract the journal. I knew it was Emil!"

"And that set you off on this murder spree? To stop Emil's constant demands? To prevent Zac from revealing the extent of your debt to the Delrey Bank?"

"Emil was draining me dry!" Elder Mackintosh could hold it in no longer. "He betrayed me! And young Garber didn't understand, would not listen to me. He wanted me to confess my guilt at the next Prayer Meeting, to ask for forgiveness. But how to forgive what cannot be helped? I had to act."

"You went to Entertainment Row with the rest of the group, but did not accompany them to Pegeen's. Instead, you waited outside until you saw a gang of Pangkoti hardbodies on the strut, looking for trouble. You sent them to Pegeen's, then you waited until Emil left.

"You followed him all the way to Fishmarket, crept up the stairs, and waited for him to send his lad out of the room for water. Then you went into his room and used the cord around your neck...watch out!"

Atterson leaped away as Mackintosh whipped the braided string out of his collar. He must have been maddened with rage, to think he could get away with violence in that crowded room.

Atterson's guards went after him. He shook them off and lunged at me, hands extended.

"I'll kill you!"

I dodged, sending him sprawling into Hunt's huge desk. He made another attempt. It took Atterson and both her Guards to get his arms behind his back and pin them with regulation binders. They propped him up with his back to the door.

"That's him!" came a shrill voice. "That's the djinn! That's the one who got Emil!"

iv

Basher loomed up behind Jakki. "I found him," he announced. "He was on his way to the docks, ready to sail back to Pangkot."

"Or to one of the villages at the mouth of the estuary," I said. "But he's here now, and I have one more strand to unwind before all this is settled.

"I understand about Emil, Elder Mackintosh, but Zac? He was your own find, you sponsored him. He trusted you. There's a witness who saw someone meet him at the carrier…that was you, wasn't it? And you killed him."

By this time, Mackintosh must have felt he had to explain himself not just to me but to the rest of the Contramonters.

"He first came to me to tell me he'd seen me with one of the Delrey mechs, and asked if it was part of the negotiations. I explained that away easily enough. Then he expressed his doubts about Junior Banker Delrey. He didn't understand why he should attract such attention, and didn't know whether or not he should respond. And he was worried, he said, because he was both attracted and repelled by those advances."

"And you were terrified, because if he responded to s Gyorgi he'd put you in a very difficult position," I

243

finished for him. "Temptation, sin—and all for what? A few minutes in a place like Vassily's?"

"I couldn't let him go to Elder Pinkney with what he knew," Elder Mackintosh whined. "It wasn't just taking payment from the Delrey Bank. Master Banker Delrey knew about me and Emil. I'd met Emil at one of the Delrey soirees. If I didn't work with the Delrey Bank, all would be discovered. I could not face that."

"So, you used the same technique on him as you did on Emil and shoved him over the railing. You hoped the tide would carry him away, or that he'd be written off as one more drunken student who fell—an accident. It nearly worked, too, but Dark One Kelvin has sharp eyes, and you didn't reckon on the vines holding Zac down so the tide couldn't get to him."

Fee M'Farr had listened to all this quietly and now he had his say.

"I told you this wasn't one of my people. None of them would be so careless. Leaving the body to be found by chance? Not checking the tides? Stupid!" He waved a hand in dismissal. "And cooking the books? Careless! My Swindlers would have done a better job.

"I'm done here. My man Brutus had nothing to do with Emil or Zac, and that's proven." He gave Mackintosh one more look of utter disdain. "Next time, hire a professional."

On his way out, he stopped to have a good look at Jakki.

"I know all about your gang of street lizards. I started the same way. You're good, you're fast, but you're small-time. You think you can take me on? Try in ten years, youngster. Until then, keep your lizards in check. Or hook up with the Guild, and learn the right way to do things."

"You wait, Old Man!" Jakki shouted. "I'll be after you, you just wait!"

"Not if I get you first."

Atterson sprang between them. "Take your business outside, and keep it between you. One Merchant's War is enough!"

Fee and Jakki glared at each other. Then Fee laughed.

"I like your style, Lizard. Come see me. Maybe we can work something out."

Jakki glowered at M'Farr's broad back as he made his way out, with Ratty close behind him.

Hunt took over again.

"Captain Atterson, I leave the rest to you. You have your murderer. Take him to detention, get him before the magistrate. He has been identified, he has confessed."

"I'm not bound by the Regulations of Lorr!" Mackintosh insisted.

"Elder Pinkney, what is the penalty for murder in Contramont?" I asked.

"Death!" he proclaimed.

"And in Lorr?"

Atterson answered, "A life in the mines."

"Your choice," I told Mackintosh. "If I were you, I'd stick with Lorr. He's all yours, Captain."

Atterson's squad took charge. Mackintosh was done, either way, and it was no longer my concern.

"Jakki," I said, "are you satisfied? I've fulfilled the terms of our contract, I've found the one who did for Emil."

"He'll be punished, one way or another." Jakki paused. "I'm sorry about…what happened. Next time, I'll think first."

"There won't be a next time," I warned him. "Make the deal with M'Farr. Learn from him. He's been around a long time, and he's not going to let you or anyone else unseat him. And you owe me one jacket and a pair of shoes."

Jakki slithered out of Basher's grip, and made for the door. Atterson intercepted him.

"Not so fast. I want to know more about these street lizards."

The two of them went off, probably to Detention. Jakki was about to learn at first hand just how pervasive Admin could be.

The Contramont Miners sat in stunned silence, staring at each other. Their chief negotiator had been revealed as a liar, a cheat, and worse. Their most promising boffin was gone. They were adrift in a place they didn't understand.

Elder Pinkney spoke first. "Independent Eye Hunt, have you nothing else to say?"

"I have fulfilled my contract," Hunt pronounced. "You asked me to uncover the missing funds. I have discovered who took them, but I regret to say, they will remain missing. I do not think the Temples of Mata Diva and Buda-Ganesha will return what Licensee Emil do-

246

nated, and the clothing he bought has already been appropriated by his friends."

"There's also the journal," I pointed out. "My contract was with Boffin Zac Garber. Now he's gone, who owns the journal? And what do you want to do with its contents?"

Elder Pinkney scowled. "The journal must not be made public. Its contents must remain unknown. Destroy it."

"That would be a pity," Hunt said. "The process for extracting coal oil may be quite lucrative, given the right apparatus."

"If it is so obvious, someone else will doubtless discover it," Elder Kennington decided. "On the other hand, the more...personal...material is far too dangerous to be revealed. I leave the journal in your hands, Eye Hunt. In my opinion, you have fulfilled your contract. That is enough. May you have a long life."

"We must find an advocate and remove Elder Mackintosh from Detention," Elder Pinkney decided. "Before he reveals too much about the negotiations."

"The negotiations with the Delrey Bank are at an end," Elder Kennington stated firmly, not daring to look at the Delreys.

Vernor sat rigid with disdain; Gyorgi slumped in his chair.

"There are other banks. I do not wish to see you again, Master Banker Delrey."

He stalked out, followed by Elder Pinkney.

That left Master Banker Delrey and Independent Eye Hunt staring each other down.

"Are you satisfied, Julian?" Vernor spat. "Have you had your petty revenge?"

"Not petty, and not revenge, Vernor," she told him. "Call it...recompense. I am not pleased, not at all. I take no satisfaction in destroying an institution like the Delrey Bank. Fortunately, there is one more Delrey, espoused to someone with more sense and a better ethic than either of you. Devon will undoubtedly take up the slack when you and Gyorgi go...elsewhere."

She waved a hand. "You never did grasp that underhanded tactics never lead to a good end. I strongly suspect you will have a visit from Security Chief Regina Polaris, on behalf of the Administration Financial Section, quite soon. You had better prepare for a thorough audit of the Delrey Bank's assets."

"Including your investment in the airship venture," I added. "That was your undoing, wasn't it? You had to get control of the Contramont mines to make up for that loss."

Vernor's face revealed nothing. He sat in stony silence for a minute or two, then said, "Investments do not always work out as planned. Unfortunately, the airships proved to be more of a financial burden than we expected.

"The scheme involved more than the mere construction of the ships. There were political complications. The mines would have provided funding, shored up our investment..." His voice trailed off. "I did not know Liaison Mackintosh was so unstable. I had no idea he would resort to such extreme measures to protect his reputation in Contramont."

"But he did, and you must bear some of the blame," Hunt said. "You may remove yourself from my presence, Vernor. I do not wish to contaminate myself and my colleagues with your evasions." She waved at Reg. "Remove them."

There was nothing more to say. The two Delreys slunk out. Reg, Basher, and I were left with Hunt.

"You have been very clever, Pola Drach. Quite satisfactory."

High praise from the Brain!

v

An hour or so later, I sat with Basher and Reg in Basher's favorite corner of Smokey Joe's. Basher was drinking jack, Reg and I stuck with brew.

"I'm still trying to sort it all out," Reg said. "The Brain got part of it right. She's known Vernor Delrey since before the Merchant's War, and she knows how he operates, so she worked out the part about the Contramont Miners and their negotiations.

"It was all a matter of coin. The Delrey Bank's in trouble, and the Contramont Mines would get them out of it if the Delreys could control the profits. Vernor Delrey wanted to get the mines by controlling the negotiator. He must have found out about Elder Mackintosh's little secret…"

"That he liked playmates of his own gender," I said. "Not something they allow in Contramont.

Basher snorted his disdain for religious restrictions. "Who cares who futters who? Whose business is it of anyone but the ones in the bed?"

"It matters in Contramont," I reminded him. "And so Mackintosh had to keep his urges secret. Until Vernor came along, recognized a kindred spirit and threw Emil into Mackintosh's path, with orders to keep him amused. Which Emil did, until he decided to take a part in the game himself."

"Game?" Basher asked through a fog of jack.

I went on. "Master Banker Vernor Delrey uses people like pieces on his board, or cards on the table. Only thing is, people don't always act like board pieces or playing cards. Emil was the wild card in the game.

"Vernor used Emil to get to Mackintosh, then Emil used Mackintosh for his own aims, which wasn't part of Vernor's plans. Jakki wanted something different from all of them. People!" I had to laugh into my brew. "No one wants what the other wants, and no one cares. What a mess!"

Basher nodded. "What I don't understand is why it took so long for the Contys to get wise to what Mackintosh was up to."

Reg took over the narration.

"The Contramont miners weren't worried until last fall, when they started getting notices from suppliers that their accounts were in arrears. That's when they started to question their representatives in Pangkot and South

Coast, and finally came to Lorr to have it out with Mackintosh.

"Eye Hunt got the reports from the Transport Guild tracing shipments of ore from Contramont. Sure enough, payments were really messed up. Mackintosh must have been siphoning off the funds for at least two years, maybe more, to pay for his little playmates. First in Pangkot, then here in Lorr."

"Is Pangkot where he learned to use the cord?" I had wondered about that.

"He was the Contramont rep there before he got here," Reg said. "That's where he must have picked up the technique. He's not as soft as he looks. All that bulk is muscle, not flab."

"He didn't need the cord, he could have used his hands, but I guess he worried that something could be traced back to him. The Dark Ones attached to the Guards have a reputation for finding things no one else can."

Basher jumped back in. "So, he tried to frame Brutus, but Brutus wasn't about to be taken without a fight. Whose bright idea was it to get Brutus involved, anyway?"

"That had to be Vernor," I guessed. "Brutus had been one of Selva Delrey's finds, straight off the boat from Pankgot with Ishka Kunine. Vernor could be sure Brutus would do what he was told."

"He did. Only, he took his time about it. And by then, Mackintosh had already done for Emil." Basher took another swig of jack.

Reg tried to sort it all out. "So, Mackintosh comes to Lorr from Pangkot. He meets with Master Banker Vernor Delrey. He gets invited to one of the Delrey soirees. Then what happens?"

"Emil happens." I sighed. "True love…or maybe lust? Whatever it was, Mackintosh had it for Emil. He thought he'd bought Emil out and set him up for himself, but Emil was still Vernor's creature, still in the sex trade, not just with Mackintosh but with others, including Gorgeous Gyorgi. And then…?"

"Mackintosh got caught." Basher snickered. "Zac saw him accepting a payoff from someone in Delrey livery,"

"And Boffin Zac might have been young and naïve, but he wasn't stupid," I said. "He knew about the negotiations, he knew the Delrey Bank was not the miners' friend. He questioned Elder Mackintosh about what he'd seen because he wanted to be reassured about his mentor. He had no way of knowing about Mackintosh's personal life, of course. But Elder Mackintosh thought he did."

"And he wanted to keep the Delreys happy," Basher added. "So, he sent Zac off to Pegeen's with the rest of the Conty party."

"There's only one part of this crazy chain of events I don't understand," Reg said. "How did Mackintosh know Emil would be at Pageen's?"

"You heard him. Vernor told him," I said. "It would be just like Vernor to dangle Emil in front of Mackintosh. Gyorgi told Vernor about the journal, and Vernor used Emil to seduce Zac. I was guessing about Mackintosh setting off the hardbodies to bust up the fun and games at Pegeen's, but it makes sense. He wanted to get Zac out of there as soon as Emil got the journal, and he wanted Emil out of there so he could follow him to somewhere private and finish him off."

"But you were right," Basher said. "I found the hardbodies who raided Pegeen's. They thought it was good fun, taking Conty coin to spoil a Conty party. I can identify Mackintosh as the one who pointed them at the Pleasure Palace."

"And as soon as Emil got the journal, he left, notifying the Guards on his way past the bridge that there was trouble at Pegeen's." I finished the sorry tale. "Only, Elder Mackintosh was waiting, somewhere between Entertainment Row and Fishmarket. He followed Emil home, lurked in the shadows behind the house until he saw Jakki leave…" I let the rest dangle.

"And hoped everyone would just let it go—one more joyboy less in Lorr. Who cares?" Basher finished his drink.

"I care," I said. "There aren't many of us humans left in the universe. As far as anyone knows, we're it. Two ships left Old Earth carrying as many humans as they could. Maybe the third ship also took off, but it never got here. Every human life on New Earth is important, even one as venal as Vernor Delrey's or as unthinking as Elder Mackintosh's."

Reg and Basher stared at me. I don't usually let my feelings show this way. It must have been the brew.

"So, Pola, how did you put it together?" Reg waved a server down for another round.

"Timing, mostly," I said. "If Zac wasn't done by Brutus, then who? After that, it was like one of those puzzles in the mags. A bunch of dots on the page, and if you connect them, they make a picture. I knew there was a Contramonter connected with Emil, and the 'djinn' Jakki saw could have been a Conty—big, with a beard covering his face.

"The others were accounted for. Among the males without alibis, the only one who fit the description was Mackintosh. Pinckney is too short, Kennington is too thin. Neither of them has a beard that covers his whole face.

"It was the Delrey connection that was missing, and Vernor gave me that by grabbing me off the street and trying to scare me into backing away. It only made me look closer at him."

"What's going to happen to the poor Conty sod?" Basher wanted to know.

"He gets his choice, death in the mines or death in the mountains," I said. "I suspect the Delrey Bank will get taken into the Vikk sphere of influence. Not my problem; let Admin Security and Finance sort it out." I stood up, a little unsteadily. "It's been an interesting case, friends, but I've had enough. I have a plant that needs some loving care."

"I'll see you back to your digs," Reg offered.

He found us a pedi-shaw, got me back to Food Alley, and let me off in front of Fletcher's. As he helped me down, I put my arms around his neck. We almost kissed, but he took my arms down and stepped back.

"It's not going to happen, is it." I made it a statement, not a question.

"You're a colleague and a good friend," he said. "Better to leave it that way."

I shrugged. "You're right. Thank the Brain for the entertainment and the good words. Stay well, Reg Bonwit."

I went up the stairs to my rooms. I was bone-tired, and the meds from the Temple were starting to wear off; but I still had my evening chores. I watered Ficus, fed it bone-meal and clet-powder, and stroked its leaves.

Two more little green shoots meant Ficus was healing. I only hoped I would.

vii

And that, you'd think, would be that. But there were consequences. There always are.

A notice went up on Post Three: the Delrey Bank was being reorganized under the supervision of the Administration Financial Department. Devon Delrey and his spouse Kaisrin Vikk would become nominal heads of the business, empowered to make decisions regarding disbursement of funds.

The Contramont Miners Trade Delegation announced the favorable terms of their agreement with the Administration regarding funding for a new refinery, one that would use a revolutionary new process to extract coal essence out of previously discarded rock from old mines.

The Garber Process was hailed as a great breakthrough that could extend the life of played-out mines. Boffins rejoiced, while conservationists railed against further exploitation of the planet and destruction of the atmosphere of New Earth.

Post Six had a flurry of announcements and speculation concerning the whereabouts of Master Banker Vernor Delrey and Junior Banker Gyorgi Delrey. Vernor supposedly was "taking a brief respite" from the business world, retreating to one of the Delrey lodges in the Mineral Mountains. Gyorgi was on an extended tour of Delrey holdings in Pangkot and South Coast, reportedly to end at Port Chicago, where he would be installed as caretaker of the Delrey Bank.

Those of Jakki's street lizards who were willing to take instruction in the fine arts of thievery were accepted into the Guild of Forgers, Assassins, Thieves, and Swindlers as apprentice Thieves, under Junior Thief Jakki's supervision. Fee M'Farr saw to it they had a dormitory and regular meals. Most of them took the offer. Those who didn't were hounded out of Lorr to Flatlands, where they caused great misery among the small shopkeepers.

Jake and Holly rejoiced to see the fad for kilts fade with the disgrace of Gorgeous Gyorgi and his cronies. Jake launched a new line of boiler suits in the same multicolored cloth as the kilts. They were very popular with the young and trim, not so flattering to anyone else.

I decided to avail myself of Zeta's services whenever I had to leave the office. She became my unofficial drone.

Ficus put out more twigs, grew more leaves, thrived on bone-meal and clet-powder, and gave me extra pheromones as a reward.

I decided to say nothing about the creature in the river. It had set me free, and I did the same for it—debt paid. No point in trying to find it again, or hand it over to boffins for study. Whatever it was, it was better off on its own, without human interference.

The Brain was gracious enough to share some of her fee from the Contramont Miners with Basher and me. I used my bit to buy a new leather jacket with a fancy zip-fastener and a warm wooly lining.

Winter was coming, and I wanted to be prepared.

END

ACKNOWLEDGEMENTS

Thanks must go to:

John Betancourt and Claudia Copupe, who let me take over their sandbox.

Eileen Watkins, Beta-reader extraordinaire, who did a bang-up editing job.

Liz Burton, who gave me the title and let me take it from there.

ABOUT THE AUTHOR

ROBERTA ROGOW got her start writing for *Star Trek* Fanzines in the mid-1970's. She mostly writes historical fiction, although she sometimes twists the history. Her previous series have taken readers to Victorian London, Gilded Age New York City, and an alternate Manhattan settled by Spanish Moors instead of Dutch traders.

Roberta spent 37 years as a children's librarian in New Jersey. She retired in 2008.and now spends her time going to science fiction and mystery conventions when she is not writing mysteries or singing filk (speculative fiction-themed folk music).

ABOUT THE ARTIST

JENNIFER GIVNER is a book cover artist and graphic designer with more than fifteen years' experience in cover design. She illustrated the very first ebook coloring book, *Double Dip Penguin Surprise: The Coloring Book*, which was carried in Barnes and Noble's NY flagship store in 2000, along with the cover for the accompanying children's book, *Double Dip Penguin Surprise*. She was featured in a six-month West Coast signing tour that was covered by Cosmo Space TV Japan.

Her cover artwork has been showcased in a variety of media including *Time* magazine, *Wired* magazine, NPR, SiriusXM, WOAI radio, BlogTalkRadio, and *Inside Sports Fishing* magazine. In 2008, she designed the program and website for the stage play *A Breach of the Peace* starring Ed Asner. All proceeds from the performances benefited Habitat for Humanity of Greater Los Angeles.